S. Hrg. 106–362

PROSTATE CANCER

HEARING

BEFORE A
SUBCOMMITTEE OF THE
COMMITTEE ON APPROPRIATIONS
UNITED STATES SENATE

ONE HUNDRED SIXTH CONGRESS

FIRST SESSION

SPECIAL HEARING

Printed for the use of the Committee on Appropriations

Available via the World Wide Web: http://www.access.gpo.gov/congress/senate

U.S. GOVERNMENT PRINTING OFFICE

59–317 cc　　　　　WASHINGTON : 2000

For sale by the U.S. Government Printing Office
Superintendent of Documents, Congressional Sales Office, Washington, DC 20402
ISBN 0–16–060204–1

COMMITTEE ON APPROPRIATIONS

TED STEVENS, Alaska, *Chairman*

THAD COCHRAN, Mississippi
ARLEN SPECTER, Pennsylvania
PETE V. DOMENICI, New Mexico
CHRISTOPHER S. BOND, Missouri
SLADE GORTON, Washington
MITCH McCONNELL, Kentucky
CONRAD BURNS, Montana
RICHARD C. SHELBY, Alabama
JUDD GREGG, New Hampshire
ROBERT F. BENNETT, Utah
BEN NIGHTHORSE CAMPBELL, Colorado
LARRY CRAIG, Idaho
KAY BAILEY HUTCHISON, Texas
JON KYL, Arizona

ROBERT C. BYRD, West Virginia
DANIEL K. INOUYE, Hawaii
ERNEST F. HOLLINGS, South Carolina
PATRICK J. LEAHY, Vermont
FRANK R. LAUTENBERG, New Jersey
TOM HARKIN, Iowa
BARBARA A. MIKULSKI, Maryland
HARRY REID, Nevada
HERB KOHL, Wisconsin
PATTY MURRAY, Washington
BYRON L. DORGAN, North Dakota
DIANNE FEINSTEIN, California
RICHARD J. DURBIN, Illinois

STEVEN J. CORTESE, *Staff Director*
LISA SUTHERLAND, *Deputy Staff Director*
JAMES H. ENGLISH, *Minority Staff Director*

SUBCOMMITTEE ON LABOR, HEALTH AND HUMAN SERVICES, AND EDUCATION, AND RELATED AGENCIES

ARLEN SPECTER, Pennsylvania, *Chairman*

THAD COCHRAN, Mississippi
SLADE GORTON, Washington
JUDD GREGG, New Hampshire
LARRY CRAIG, Idaho
KAY BAILEY HUTCHISON, Texas
TED STEVENS, Alaska
JON KYL, Arizona

TOM HARKIN, Iowa
ERNEST F. HOLLINGS, South Carolina
DANIEL K. INOUYE, Hawaii
HARRY REID, Nevada
HERB KOHL, Wisconsin
PATTY MURRAY, Washington
DIANNE FEINSTEIN, California
ROBERT C. BYRD, West Virginia
(Ex officio)

Professional Staff

BETTILOU TAYLOR
MARY DIETRICH
JIM SOURWINE
AURA DUNN
ELLEN MURRAY *(Minority)*

Administrative Support

KEVIN JOHNSON
CAROLE GEAGLEY *(Minority)*

CONTENTS

PROSTATE CANCER

WEDNESDAY, JUNE 16, 1999

U.S. SENATE,
SUBCOMMITTEE ON LABOR, HEALTH AND HUMAN
SERVICES, AND EDUCATION, AND RELATED AGENCIES,
COMMITTEE ON APPROPRIATIONS,
Washington, DC.

The subcommittee met at 9:34 a.m., in room SD–192, Dirksen Senate Office Building, Hon. Arlen Specter (chairman) presiding.

Present: Senators Specter, Cochran, Stevens, and Feinstein.

DEPARTMENT OF HEALTH AND HUMAN SERVICES

NATIONAL INSTITUTES OF HEALTH

STATEMENTS OF:
HAROLD VARMUS, M.D., DIRECTOR
RICHARD KLAUSNER, M.D., DIRECTOR, NATIONAL CANCER INSTI-
TUTE

NONDEPARTMENTAL WITNESSES

STATEMENTS OF:
CHRISTOPHER LOGOTHETIS, M.D., CHAIRMAN AND PROFESSOR OF
CLINICAL CANCER, DEPARTMENT OF MEDICAL ONCOLOGY, UNI-
VERSITY OF TEXAS
ROBERT DOLE, FORMER U.S. SENATOR
MICHAEL MILKEN, FOUNDER AND CHAIRMAN, CapCURE, ASSOCIA-
TION FOR THE CURE OF CANCER OF THE PROSTATE
JOE TORRE, MANAGER, NEW YORK YANKEES

OPENING STATEMENT OF SENATOR ARLEN SPECTER

Senator SPECTER. The hearing of the Appropriations Subcommittee on Labor, Health and Human Services, and Education will now proceed. Our subject today is on prostate cancer. We will be reviewing the funding and the work of the National Institutes of Health and the National Cancer Institute.

We have a very distinguished array of visitors today: Dr. Harold Varmus, Director of NIH; Dr. Richard Klausner, Director of the National Cancer Institute; Dr. Christopher Logothetis, chairman and professor of Clinical Cancer Research at the University of Texas; Senator Robert Dole, former Senate majority leader; Mr. Michael Milken, founder and chairman of the Association for the Cure of Cancer of the Prostate; and Mr. Joe Torre, manager of the New York Yankees.

The issue of research on funding is one of enormous importance and it is front and center in the Congress of the United States today. There is a consensus that research is necessary and that the funding ought to be provided, and when the sense of the Senate resolution was voted on not too long ago, it passed 98 to nothing to double research for NIH over 5 years.

Those were the druthers, the preferences. But when the time came to put up the dollars, the votes were not there. Three years ago, Senator Harkin and I authored an initiative to add a billion dollars which was defeated 63 to 37. We sharpened our pencils and found the money by establishing priorities in our existing funds.

Two years ago a similar effort was made and again we were defeated, 57 to 42, but we were moving up. Last year again, we lost 52 to 48, but we were able to add some $2 billion to the total of NIH, and that has been reflected in the funding which has been provided for the Cancer Institute, which for fiscal year 1999 was $2.93 billion, a $375.9 million increase over fiscal year 1998.

But our work is cut out for us this year if we are to be able to find the funding. We have not been able to move ahead with the processing, so-called "markup," of the subcommittee bill here because of the caps and limitations, and we are struggling now to find the funds.

This subcommittee is committed and determined to do its utmost to find increased funding for NIH, and we have again targeted an increase of $2 billion. Whether that will occur remains to be seen. But this is a dedicated crowd today, a dedicated audience, which can play a significant role in helping put the political pressure on Congress to get this kind of funding, and these kinds of high visibility hearings have a very significant effect.

My own personal view is that it is unthinkable in a country as wealthy as ours not to fund all the meritorious applications for research, that is not to fund them all if they are meritorious, and the decision ought to be made on really if they are worthwhile, not whether we have the money to do it. This is a rich and powerful country and we have a Federal budget of $1.7 trillion and there is no higher priority than health.

Just this week it was brought home to me. My former executive director in Philadelphia has a daughter who is 13. I was there at her birth. She has lymphoma, and fortunately she has a good prognosis. My chief of staff yesterday told me that his 14-year-old nephew has such a serious case of cancer that they are going to be excising his shoulder blade.

I look at my three grandchildren and I look at my own PSA score and I see the people who are here today, prostate cancer survivors, and say that we ought to be funding every last research grant which is meritorious. We can afford to do it and we cannot afford not to do it.

Senator Dole has been a leader in this field for a very long time. In 1991, he had a prostate cancer operation and he came back to the Republican Caucus. We were assembled for our Tuesday lunch and he said: "I just had a successful prostate operation; it strikes one man out of nine; you eight fellows are safe." Then he pointed to Ted Stevens and he said: "Ted just had a prostate operation, successful, and you eight fellows are safe."

Then he turned and looked at Strom and he said: "Strom, you are too old to get prostate cancer." [Laughter.]

Bob and I are from the same little town in Kansas, so I am permitted to steal one joke a month, to replay one of his stories.

But he has been a tremendous leader in the field. He has made a suggestion which I think is an excellent one, that everybody in the room who is a prostate cancer survivor should stand, if you would, please. [Men stand.]

Thank you all very much. Congratulations to you.

You can be a model for others.

I want to turn now to our two very distinguished research scientists: Dr. Harold Varmus, Director of the National Institutes of Health; and Dr. Richard Klausner, Director of the National Cancer Institute. In the appropriations, where we have very materially increased NIH funding, I must candidly say that there are questions raised by my colleagues as to whether the NIH can really use these funds effectively and whether they are using them efficiently. The subcommittee sent Dr. Varmus a letter recently asking for details on their expenditures, what they are doing with the funds.

In looking to next year, we have examined, and we will be looking at it further, a spreadsheet as to where these funds are going to go. Those are very important questions to be answered because too often major Federal agencies turn up with big deficiencies, and all you need is one big deficiency and then forget about the funding. There are so many places to fund. It has to be done and it has to be done right.

We have had a fairly sharp response. Again, candidly and openly, I want to put all the cards up on the table on the problems as well as the successes. But when we had to cancel an earlier scheduled hearing on prostate cancer because the report which was originally scheduled to be released on April 22 was not released—and it is going to be released today—we got two letters from prostate cancer community leaders expressing concern to Dr. Varmus that the missed deadlines exemplified the NIH's "neglect and indifference" to cancer sufferers and "abruptly terminated its commitment" to prostate cancer sufferers.

So the kind of a sense of urgency which we have has to be recognized at all times. We are constantly beset with a variety of people, well intentioned sufferers from one malady or another, what want to know why their particular ailment is not getting more funding, and they can always find one to point to, which on a per capita basis, is getting more.

The subcommittee and the full committee and the Congress have stayed away from our judgment. We want to leave it to your judgments, the medical judgments and the peer judgments, as to what ought to be funded.

SUMMARY STATEMENT OF DR. HAROLD VARMUS

We turn now to Dr. Harold Varmus, who has been Director of the NIH since November of 1993. At the University of California at San Francisco he won the Nobel Prize for his work on the causative link between certain genes and cancer. A graduate of Amherst College, Harvard University, and the Columbia Medical School.

Thank you for your contribution, Dr. Varmus. Thank you for joining us today. The floor is yours.

Dr. VARMUS. Thank you, Senator Specter.

Senator SPECTER. Our rules provide for a 5-minute green light, 1-minute yellow light, and a red light. So to the extent we can stay within those time limits it would be appreciated.

Dr. VARMUS. Senator, thank you. I will be very brief. I am going to turn over most of my time to Dr. Klausner, who, as the Director of NCI, coordinates the trans-NIH efforts on this particular problem, prostate cancer. But I did want to make a few comments before yielding the microphone to him.

First, I want to thank you for holding this hearing on this very important scientific and medical topic. It allows us to show a specific example of how the NIH can respond with increased research activity against a major public health threat, especially when we are equipped with the increased funds which your Committee has provided for us and when we are supported by the remarkable progress that has been made in our understanding of cancer at the genetic, cell biological and physiological level over the last several years.

It also allows us to illustrate how research activities can be coordinated within a major institute like the NCI and across the several NIH institutes that are active in research against prostate cancer. As you will see in your reading of the report, there are nine institutes and centers that have some involvement in prostate cancer research; but for the most part their involvement is relatively minor compared to the activity of the NCI, which funds over 85 percent of prostate cancer-specific research at the NIH.

I want to commend the NCI in particular for a thorough planning process that has been ongoing now for at least 2 to 3 years, bringing in a large array of activists, scientists, patients, and others.

I also want to apologize for any delay in the issuance of the report. This was not a delay that had any impact on our execution of the scientific programs, but represented a misapprehension by us about how much time it would take to get the report through the various clearing processes at the Department and OMB and elsewhere in order to deliver the report in a finished, cleared manner to you at the hearing.

But let me restate that we are sorry that any of the prostate cancer patients felt that this represented any lack of commitment on our part or any delay in the scientific agenda. Neither was true, although that impression is clearly understandable. I hope that with the issuance of the report today and our report on what has been achieved in prostate cancer in the last couple of years those who are most concerned about this disease will be at least partially reassured.

I again thank you for holding the hearing, and, would like to turn the proceedings over to Dr. Klausner.

SUMMARY STATEMENT OF DR. RICHARD KLAUSNER

Senator SPECTER. We turn now to Dr. Richard Klausner. Appointed Director of the National Cancer Institute in August of 1995, he has served as Chief of Cell Biology and Metabolism

Branch of the National Institute of Child Health and Human Development. Undergraduate degree from Yale, a medical degree from Duke, and postgraduate work at Harvard.

Thank you for all you have done, Dr. Klausner. We look forward to your testimony.

Dr. KLAUSNER. Thank you, Senator Specter, for both having this hearing and providing the leadership and support that has allowed us to, as I think I will show you, act with the sense of urgency that we all feel is needed to make progress against prostate cancer. I am particularly pleased to appear before you today to describe our response to the congressional request to develop a plan and a professional judgment estimate of the scientific opportunities in prostate cancer.

Prostate cancer is the single most common form of cancer of men in the United States. This year alone, NCI predicts there will be 179,000 new diagnoses of prostate cancer and about 37,000 men will die of the disease. It exacts a particularly devastating toll in the African American community, with 50 percent increased incidence and a twofold increase in mortality compared to white Americans.

But this catalogue of prostate cancer statistics does little to convey the real fear and pain and uncertainty experienced by men when they are diagnosed with prostate cancer. Despite advances over the past decades, currently our treatments for prostate cancer are inadequate. The side effects of treatment are unacceptable and troubling questions remain about the efficacy of early detection for this disease. Every day too many men in the United States hear the life-changing words, "You have prostate cancer." Too many men are faced with the agonizing decision of how to treat their prostate cancer, and too many men are dying too young of this disease.

PROSTATE CANCER RESEARCH PLAN

Dr. Varmus said nine NIH Institutes are involved in this prostate cancer research plan. The NCI is the lead Institute, responsible for the majority of the research, and we participate in and help coordinate all of these activities. This morning I am going to focus on the NCI activities.

The request for this report in last year's appropriations bill came at a propitious time in NCI's internal planning and implementation process. Over 2 years ago, we initiated a prostate cancer review process, bringing together scientists, clinicians and advocates, challenging all of us together to review our current prostate cancer research portfolio, to develop a prioritized set of questions that needed to be answered, to identify resources that needed to be developed, and to provide a vision to chart a course for prostate cancer research.

This is the report and we are happy to make it available to the Committee. It has been very helpful to have this report so that we have a set of priorities as we move forward with increased investments.

The report being presented today is a two-part plan for research in prostate cancer. First, the current fiscal year 1999 budget commits a 63-percent increase over fiscal year 1998, for a projected total of $141.5 million this year for NCI and $180 million for NIH for prostate cancer. Second, we have developed a professional judgment estimate covering the following four fiscal years.

But we have already this year embarked on an aggressive prostate cancer research agenda based upon this several years of planning, and it is this aggressive agenda that will lay the groundwork for future efforts as described in the report. The report lays out clear priorities.

PROSTATE CANCER CLINICAL TRIALS

Seventy percent of the targeted dollars would be directed to clinical and translational research, with the opportunity to rapidly, with near-term outcomes, affect the experience of men with prostate cancer. Let me illustrate this with a few examples. In the areas of clinical trials for patients with prostate cancer, we have set out explicit goals to test new approaches and new agents aimed at a variety of clinical situations that men face. We have established a novel program we call Quick Trials to provide a rapid and efficient way to move new ideas for therapeutic interventions out of the laboratory into phase one and phase two clinical trials for prostate cancer.

This program will greatly increase the critical early phase clinical trials carried out at cancer centers around the country. The NCI's goals this year are to increase the number of patients participating in early clinical trials in prostate cancer by two to threefold and to initiate 10 to 15 new trials in the first year of this Quick Trials program.

In addition, the NCI's Cancer Therapy Evaluation Program will initiate approximately 35 new phase one and two trials in prostate cancer, with over 25 novel drugs, agents, or combinations, many of which have not been used before but show promise in the laboratory, directed against a number of particularly promising molecular targets and mechanisms, which is what we have to move toward.

The targets include: angiogenesis and metastasis, the process by which cancer induces new blood vessels, invades those blood vessels, and is spread through the body; targets against growth factors and their receptors, which mediate the growth and the survival of prostate cancer cells; and targets against genes whose products are specifically expressed in normal prostate and prostate cancer cells, thus allowing us to specifically target a variety of killing modalities.

In these trials we will test novel small molecule drugs, specific antibodies, vaccines, targeted gene therapy, targeted radiation sensitizers, and others.

Now, compared to the level of effort in 1998, this plan already more than doubles the number of early clinical trials initiated in prostate cancer in 1999. This year, we will additionally activate up to ten new multi-center phase three clinical trials in prostate cancer that will attempt to optimize hormonal approaches and move forward with important new chemotherapeutic approaches for the most common clinical presentations of the disease, including adjuvant therapy in the setting of primary surgical or radiation treatment. In fact, in recent clinical trials we have been able to see the first reduction in mortality from more aggressive regional prostate cancer with this combination of adjuvant therapy with radiation.

We will look at neo-adjuvant therapy, treatment after hormone therapy, treatment in the setting of rising PSA levels after definitive local therapy, and, importantly, new treatments for advanced and metastatic disease.

With this initial ramp up in clinical trials, and contingent upon overall funding levels, we estimate the ability to double again the number of new phase three trials initiated over the following 4 years. The agents entering these trials are new and have shown significant promise in early phase trials against prostate cancer, and these early results bolster our hope that we can rapidly expand the currently very limited selection of therapies that are available for men with prostate cancer with advanced or recurrent disease.

The NCI is also engaged in a major restructuring of its clinical trials system to expand, speed and improve clinical trials. We have been working this past year very productively with CapCURE to develop and deploy a common data element system for protocol authoring, trial simplification, monitoring, reporting, and analysis.

RAPID ACCESS TO INTERVENTION DEVELOPMENT PROGRAM

We have initiated a new program which we call the RAID program, creating a virtual drug development system for the Nation that enables investigators in laboratories, academia, or small business to access resources, to move molecules out of the laboratory and into new clinical trials within 12 to 24 months. This year we have already approved 25 new agents that have not been used before in patients through the RAID program, at least 5 of which are directly related to prostate cancer and the majority of which appear relevant to prostate cancer.

Over the next 5 years our goal is that 25 or more novel therapeutics relevant to prostate cancer will be brought out of the laboratory into patients through this mechanism.

HIGH PRIORITY QUESTIONS RELATED TO PROSTATE CANCER

As laid out in the report, we are addressing a number of additional high priority questions about prostate cancer, and I will quickly review that list:

First, we will be testing promising preventive agents, particularly in high risk individuals.

Second, and this is very important, we have laid out a goal to switch prostate cancer diagnosis from the way it has been done for years, looking under the microscope, to molecular diagnostics. So we will learn which prostate cancers are going to spread, which are not going to grow, which may need therapy, and how to tailor therapy to the molecular machines in each prostate cancer.

Third, we will validate current and develop new early detection markers through the newly established early detection research network. This year we will expand the critical PLCO early detection trial involving 75,000 men followed for the development of prostate cancer. We have in the last few months established an international consortium to monitor and rapidly share data on screening of prostate cancer results throughout the world.

Fourth, we will develop a National Cooperative Prostate Cancer Tissue Resource beginning this year.

Fifth, we will expand studies linking imaging, especially functional imaging, to therapy.

Sixth, we will enhance the Specialized Programs of Research Excellence in prostate cancer by expanding the numbers of programs and by linking the current three programs around the country into a national consortium.

Seventh, we will accelerate epidemiologic studies that are ongoing to attempt to systematically identify correlates of the profound geographic and population differences in prostate cancer rates.

PREPARED STATEMENT

Finally, we have laid out a program to develop new animal models, the lack of which has limited research progress in the past, that will attempt to faithfully reproduce human prostate cancer in order to better understand tumor development and spread and as a way to more rapidly test preventive and therapeutic interventions.

Senator SPECTER. Dr. Klausner, we are having two votes scheduled at 10:45. Those votes were put in the schedule long after we had scheduled this. So to the extent you could summarize, we would appreciate it.

Dr. KLAUSNER. That was the end of my statement. I appreciate the level of interest the committee has shown in prostate cancer and I am pleased to present this report, which gives a vision of our commitment and our sense of urgency that we have had for prostate cancer.

I know Dr. Varmus and I are pleased to answer any questions you or your colleagues will have.

Senator SPECTER. Well, thank you very much, Dr. Klausner.

[The statement follows:]

PREPARED STATEMENT OF RICHARD KLAUSNER

INTRODUCTION

Good morning, Senator Specter and Members of the Subcommittee. I am Richard Klausner, M.D., Director of the National Cancer Institute (NCI). I am accompanied today by Harold Varmus, M.D., Director of the National Institutes of Health (NIH).

We are pleased to appear before you today to describe our response to the Congressional request to submit (1) a report outlining activities NIH is undertaking to enhance prostate cancer research programs and (2) a report outlining NIH's professional judgment for prostate cancer research for the next five years. The Congress has also asked NIH to make prostate cancer a top priority in allocating funding increases; to accelerate spending on prostate cancer; and to consult closely with the research community.

The nature and magnitude of the burden of prostate cancer has been tracked by NCI's surveillance program, and we estimate that about 180,000 men will be newly diagnosed with prostate cancer this year and about 37,000 will die. Prostate cancer exacts a particularly devastating toll on African American men; incidence rates are substantially higher among African Americans, and mortality rates in African American men remain more than twice as high as rates in white men.

This catalogue of statistics, while accurate, does little to convey the very real pain, fear, and uncertainty experienced by every man who is diagnosed with prostate cancer. Despite advances over the past decade, our treatments for prostate cancer are inadequate, the side effects of treatment are unacceptable, and troubling questions remain about the efficacy of early detection for the disease. Every day, too many men in the United States hear the life-changing words "You have prostate cancer." Every day, too many men are faced with the agonizing decision of how to treat their prostate cancer. And every day, too many men are dying too young of this disease. The limited knowledge about the causes of prostate cancer, how to prevent it and how to successfully treat it demand a clearly articulated and adequate approach to research.

OVERVIEW

The NIH, with leadership from NCI, has aggressively sought participation from researchers, advocates, and patients in reviewing the prostate cancer research portfolio and charting a plan for a vigorous expansion of the prostate cancer research program. The initial evaluation of the research program and a broad outline of future directions were completed in August 1998 and are described in part I of the report being presented today, "Planning for Prostate Cancer Research: Expanding the Scientific Framework." The NIH efforts in coordinating a research plan for prostate cancer have focused on continuing development of a widely disseminated research program coordinated and supported by the NIH and accompanied by continuing involvement of researchers, professional societies, advocacy groups and patients. The report of the NCI-convened Prostate Cancer Progress Review Group described a nationwide program involving a significant investment in infrastructure across the nation. It is recognized that each of the 35 NCI Comprehensive Cancer Centers, geographically dispersed throughout the nation, devote significant effort to education, training, treatment and research on prostate cancer and cover the full spectrum of prevention, early diagnosis and treatment.

Part II of the report, "Planning for Prostate Cancer Research: Five Year Professional Judgment Estimates," describes prostate cancer research opportunities from 1999 through 2003. NIH has increased prostate cancer research funding significantly from a 1998 level of $114 million to a current projection of $180 million in 1999. This plan estimates that $420 million of potential research opportunities could be supported in 2003. It must be noted that this estimate is based on our assessment of scientific opportunities over the next five years, without consideration of economic constraints or other competing priorities of the NIH or the Federal government. This plan includes many efforts already initiated in 1999. Two institutes, the National Institute of Mental Health and the National Institute of Deafness and Other Communication Disorders were not previously focused on prostate research, but are now newly included in the NIH prostate efforts. Furthermore, this level of support must be integrated with other research efforts of the NIH. A total of nine institutes have important intersecting interests that contribute to the NIH prostate cancer research effort and have been consulted in the development of this plan.

NCI HIGHLIGHTS

The NCI is the lead NIH institute for prostate cancer research. The report describes a number of new NCI initiatives, projects, and mechanisms that have the potential to directly improve the quality of life of prostate cancer patients and survivors, as well as those at risk for the disease. Indeed, fully 70 percent of the research opportunities presented here are targeted at clinical or translational research that would have a direct impact on patients, survivors, and at-risk men.

The request in last year's appropriation bill for such a report came at a propitious time in NCI's internal planning and implementation processes. Before describing this plan, following are several relevant features of the NCI planning processes.

For the past 3½ years, the NCI has taken an intense three-part approach to planning. First, we established a series of blue-ribbon committees to review and propose reforms to our major venues for cancer research including clinical trials, cancer prevention, cancer control and the drug discovery and development processes. Scores of recommendations to create more effective and efficient means of making progress have or are being implemented.

Second, we established a process to evaluate areas of extraordinary opportunity with new investments and new programs that promised to capitalize on untapped, near term opportunities to make progress against cancer. These opportunities and the plans and progress made are outlined in the NCI By-Pass Budget.

Neither of these first two planning approaches are specific to cancer sites. Rather, the planning and implementation processes are specifically charged with establishing the commonality of needs across all cancer sites and to assure that the opportunities for progress are likewise implemented for all cancer sites.

Third, over two years ago, we initiated a disease-specific planning process called a progress review group or PRG. The Prostate Cancer PRG involved scores of individuals—scientists, clinicians, and advocates—and challenged the prostate cancer research community and the NCI to review our current prostate cancer research portfolio, to develop a prioritized set of questions that needed to be answered and resources that needed to be developed or applied, and provide a vision to chart a course for research and progress in prostate cancer. The PRG report was presented to the NCI last September and since then we have acted to implement a plan that we believe will fulfill the vision of progress articulated by the PRG. The PRG report, which I am pleased to provide to this committee, represents an important component of the scientific opportunities and professional judgment report which we are presenting today.

The PRG not only gave us a consensus vision of what the needs are but, importantly, greatly reinforced the premise of our other planning processes in that the vast majority of identified research needs in prostate cancer (and for breast cancer from the parallel breast cancer PRG) could be directly accommodated and accomplished through the several dozen programs already initiated as a result of our more global planning.

In all three of our planning phases we have involved a variety of members of the prostate cancer communities including researchers, clinicians and advocates. To ensure that the professional and advocacy groups were fully represented, the PRG invited the input of 32 "stakeholder" groups that represented both professional societies and advocacy groups.

The report being presented today highlights that NCI plans to spend $114.5 million on prostate cancer research in fiscal year 1999, a 63 percent increase over fiscal year 1998. NIH in total expects to spend $180 million on prostate cancer research in fiscal year 1999. At the Congress' request, we have also developed a five-year professional judgment estimate in collaboration with eight other Institutes and Centers that includes what we foresee as prostate cancer research opportunities over the following four fiscal years. If we could not be concerned with any economic constraints or other competing priorities of the NIH or the Federal government, we estimate NCI could support $340 million, and NIH in total could support $420 million worth of targeted prostate cancer research by fiscal year 2003.

We have begun, in an aggressive way, to accelerate funding for prostate cancer as reflected in the report being presented here today.

—A special section of the NCI Web site calls attention to more than 20 initiatives through which high priority areas can be addressed.

—I have met with the representatives of the prostate cancer research community, the PRG, and the leadership of professional societies, such as the American Urological Association, in order to communicate these initiatives and to enlist the research community's support in responding to these opportunities.

—Extensive outreach and advertising will alert the larger research community to these opportunities to energize their participation in this prostate cancer research program.

The scientific opportunities we project are presented in four major areas:

(1) Clinical Science—the near term direct testing of new interventions in patients or in those at risk for prostate cancer.

(2) Translational Science—moving ideas from the laboratory to the point of clinical testing.

(3) Risk, Burdens & Outcomes Science—attempting to ask critical questions about cause, the unequal levels of cancer in different populations, outcomes and survivorship.

(4) Basic research and discovery—longer term investments in gaining insight into the development and biology of prostate cancer and the development of models for study.

Priorities are identified in the report. Seventy percent of the targeted research opportunities are directed to clinical and translational research. Let me illustrate with a few examples. In the area of clinical trials for patients with prostate cancer, we need to test new approaches and new agents aimed at a variety of clinical situations. We have established "Quick Trials," a new program to provide a rapid and efficient way to move new ideas for therapeutic interventions into Phase I and II clinical trials for prostate cancer. This program has been set up in recognition of the urgent need for new types of interventions that are effective at different stages of prostate cancer, as well as the growing number of therapeutic ideas that are ready to be tested in patients.

In this type of project, where it is necessary to evaluate untested leads in the absence of preliminary data, conventional application and review procedures are not well suited. Quick Trials utilizes a process for rapid approval of early clinical trials. The NCI's goals are to increase the number of patients participating in early clinical trials by two to three-fold and to initiate 10–15 new trials through this accelerated mechanism. In addition, this year through NCI's Cancer Therapy Evaluation Program, we will initiate approximately 35 new Phase I/II trials in Prostate Cancer with agents directed against a number of particularly promising molecular targets and mechanisms. The targets include:

—angiogenesis and metastasis, the processes by which cancers induce new blood-vessel formation, invade these blood vessels, and spread throughout the body;

—growth factors and their receptors, which mediate growth signals to cancer cells; and

—tissue-specific genes expressed selectively in prostate or prostate cancer cells, thus allowing for the targeting of tumor-killing modalities to these cells.

We will test:

—Novel small molecule drugs

—Specific antibodies

—Vaccines

—Virus-based gene therapy

—Targeted radiation sensitizers

Compared to the current level of effort, this plan could more than double the number of early clinical trials in prostate cancer in the first year, with another doubling projected at the full professional judgment in the next four years.

This year, we will activate 5 new multi-center phase III clinical trials in prostate cancer that will attempt to optimize and test new hormonal and chemotherapeutic approaches for the most common clinical presentations of the disease, including:

—adjuvant therapy in the setting of primary surgical or radiation treatment;

—neo-adjuvant therapy, which has shown promising results in reducing the mortality from locally advanced prostate cancer;

—treatment after hormone therapy;

—treatment in the setting of rising PSA levels after definitive local therapy; and

—advanced disease, particularly directed at bony metastases.

With this initial ramp up in clinical trials, we project the ability to double the number again over the following four years.

We have initiated a new program creating a drug development process that enables investigators to begin clinical trials with novel molecules discovered in academic laboratories. We do this by giving academic investigators access, on a competitive basis, to NCI's preclinical drug development resources and expertise. Investigators who have molecules that hold promise for cancer treatment but without access to the development resources required for initiation of clinical studies are invited to submit applications twice a year. Those selected for support are assisted with necessary development steps to enable IND filing with the Food and Drug Administration and to begin initiation of proof-of-principle clinical trials. For fiscal year 1999, our goal is the development of three to five new therapeutic agents, each relevant to prostate cancer. Projects already approved include development of a bio-reductive compound with potential as a radio and chemosensitizer, and a gene-therapy approach that will convert inactive pro-drugs into toxic agents within prostate cancer cells. Over five years, 15 new therapeutic agents for prostate cancer could potentially be developed.

The plan covers a number of additional central questions about prostate cancer and describes potential strategies to address them. These include:

(1) Testing promising preventive agents, particularly in high risk individuals;

(2) Developing new, predictive molecular diagnostics;

(3) Validating current and new early detection markers;

(4) The linkage of imaging to therapy;

(5) Epidemiologic studies to attempt to systematically identify correlates of the profound geographic and population differences in prostate cancer rates; and

(6) Developing new animal models that faithfully reproduce human prostate cancer in order to better understand tumor development and spread, and to better test preventive and therapeutic interventions.

This plan also envisions opportunities for a four-year increment of 215 investigator-initiated research grants that target 18 areas of clinical, translational, epidemiologic and fundamental research.

The five year professional judgment report I am presenting today builds on a strong base of existing prostate cancer research including:

1. The Cancer Genome Anatomy Project (CGAP), the goals of which are to build an index of all genes that are expressed in tumors and support development of new technologies that will allow high throughput analysis of gene and protein expression as well as mutation detection. The tumor type with the highest representation in the early stages of the CGAP effort is prostate cancer. NCI has facilitated investigator collaborations of interdisciplinary studies following the recent discovery of a susceptibility gene on chromosome 1. Leads from this effort may help to clarify genetic and gene-environment interactions responsible for black-white differences in risk.

2. NCI funded (in total or in part) 246 clinical trials in prostate cancer, including 80 Phase III studies and 37 Phase II studies. NCI clinical studies in prostate cancer

have significant African-American participation. One NCI study shows that 14.7 percent of men enrolled onto NCI sponsored prostate cancer treatment trials are African American while 10.3 percent of Americans diagnosed with prostate cancer are African American.

3. NCI's ongoing Prostate Cancer Prevention Trial (PCPT) involves 18,000 healthy men over the age of 55 to determine if the drug finasteride can prevent prostate cancer.

4. NCI's ongoing Prostate, Lung, Colorectal, and Ovarian Cancer Screening Trial (PLCO) is assessing the efficacy of prostate cancer screening. New PLCO sites are being added to enhance minority patient accrual. NCI is sponsoring two trials in which "watchful waiting" is being compared in terms of outcome with surgical removal of the prostate and with radiation therapy. These trials are intended to determine if treatment of localized disease is effective.

5. NCI staff and the Department of Defense have collaborated in a study of treatment data and shown that equal treatment yields equal outcome within stage. This finding suggests that all NCI efforts to improve prevention, diagnosis and treatment of this disease benefit all patients equally. However, NCI staff analyzing SEER Program data have shown that there are tremendously differing patterns of care among black and white men with prostate cancer.

6. NCI, along with the American Cancer Society and the Centers for Disease Control and Prevention sponsored a Leadership Conference on Prostate Cancer in the African-American Community in November of 1997. Developed in cooperation with the 100 Black Men of America, the Intercultural Cancer Council, the National Black Leadership on Cancer, and the National Prostate Cancer Coalition, the conference represented a significant step toward developing a strategy for the full participation of African Americans in prostate cancer research and control.

7. In addition, NCI recently conducted a large interview-based study of prostate cancer in African Americans and whites. Analysis of the results have not thus far revealed any specific factor that could explain the racial differences in risk. However, further studies are underway, including an extensive evaluation of the role of different components of the diet.

OTHER INSTITUTES

Several NIH Institutes conduct and support research on prostate cancer and related diseases that will advance our knowledge of prostate cancer [National Institute of Diabetes and Digestive & Kidney Diseases (NIDDK); National Human Genome Research Institute (NHGRI); National Center for Research Resources; National Institute of Environmental Health Sciences (NIEHS); National Institute on Aging; National Institute of Nursing Research; National Institute of Mental Health; National Institute of Deafness and Other Communication Disorders]. These research activities are coordinated through formal and informal collaborations, interest groups, and other interactions. Following are highlights from some of these Institutes' professional judgment of potential research opportunities. A complete description of the research activities of other NIH Institutes may be found in the report, "Planning for Prostate Cancer Research."

NIDDK

The discoveries that will lead to improved therapy and ultimately prevention and cure need to be sought through a number of avenues:

—The outcome of cancer depends not just on the behavior of the tumor cell—but also on the normal surrounding cells that are not themselves cancerous. We need to know more about the normal prostate cells -B and the genes they express—in order to identify new targets for disease intervention. We also need to know more about the interactions between prostate cancer cells and bone, to understand the determinants of metastasis.

—Developmental biology is proving to be an important source of clues about disease. We need to understand the developmental program for formation of the prostate and the lineage of the cells that make up the gland.

—What is the action of androgen, the genes it controls and the mechanisms by which the hormone turns genes on and off? These are critical basic questions broadly anticipated to yield the basis for new therapeutic approaches.

—We know too little about the variation in susceptibility of different populations to the disease of the prostate. Careful monitoring of epidemiological trends in the burden of benign and malignant prostate disease is an important priority. Particularly, the enhanced susceptibility of certain racial groups to prostate cancer—and the relative protection of other groups—are phenomena that we need to understand.

—Better strategies to prevent the two feared complications of surgery on the prostate—urinary incontinence and impotence—are needed urgently. Although new surgical approaches for both benign prostatic hypertrophy and prostate cancer have reduced the rate of these complications, further progress is needed.

—Prostate cancer is a hormone responsive tumor and the major forms of treatment of advanced prostate cancer involve pharmacologic blockade of the gonadatrophin release or antagonism of the androgen receptor. There are new and emerging opportunities to improve these approaches.

NHGRI

Over the next five years, NHGRI investigators aim to identify all of the common contributing genes to hereditary susceptibility—besides HPC1 and HPCX, there is strong evidence pointing to another region of another chromosome, and other regions also contain hints of hereditary factors. As the precise genes are identified, clinical studies would be undertaken to offer genetic testing to men from high risk families, to identify those at greatest risk for life-threatening disease and design a program of surveillance to identify their cancers early enough to achieve cure. In addition, using the chip technology, the common changes in gene expression that contribute to various steps in malignant transformation would be cataloged, and used to derive new hypotheses about the molecular steps involved in prostate cancer. These would in turn suggest new and more powerful ways to treat or prevent the disease.

NIEHS

Human diseases, such as prostate cancer, are generally the consequence of both genetic susceptibility and environmental exposure. The tools of molecular genetics provide new opportunities to understand the genetic basis for individual differences in susceptibility to environmental exposure. The NIEHS is expanding its research program on genetic susceptibility to environmentally-associated diseases through a new Environmental Genome Project. Over the next five years, the Environmental Genome Project would systematically identify the allelic variants of disease susceptibility genes in the U.S. population, develop a central database of known polymorphisms for these genes, and foster population-based studies of gene- environment interaction in disease etiology. By identifying those genes and allelic variants that affect individual response to environmental toxins, we can better predict health risks and develop environmental policies to protect the most vulnerable subgroups of the population from such diseases such as prostate cancer.

The NIEHS Environmental Genome Project would be a broad, multi-center effort to identify systematically in the U.S. population the alleles of environmental disease susceptibility genes. Susceptibility genes will be chosen through a peer-reviewed process and are expected to include five broad gene classes: genes controlling the distribution and metabolism of toxicants; genes for the DNA repair pathways; genes for the cell cycle control system; cell death/differentiation genes; and, genes for signal transduction systems controlling expression of the genes in the other classes. This effort would result in the systematic identification of the polymorphisms of these genes found in the U.S. population. A central database of the polymorphisms would be made available. This database will support both functional studies of alleles and population-based studies of disease risk.

PUBLIC UNDERSTANDING

Communicating with cancer patients, individuals at high risk for cancer, the general public, and the health care community is a central component of NCI's mission and mandate. For prostate cancer, the institute communicates information to all of those groups, as well as to the cancer research community.

Materials available from NCI, including print, video, and web products, range from basic information about the disease, information about research now ongoing to improve understanding and management of the disease, and information for men about early detection and treatment options.

One of the most recent communications initiatives is a partnership with the prostate cancer advocacy organization, US TOO, to develop a national communications initiative, called Know Your Options, to better inform men and their families about the disease. The initiative is based on an information package or kit that provides a solid base of information about prostate cancer to help US TOO chapters work with their hometown media. The media, in turn, use the information provided by US TOO with the NCI imprimatur, to keep their readers, listeners, and viewers informed about the disease. The kit includes the latest medical and scientific information available, as well as information about where US TOO chapter leaders can go for more information, advice, and help.

In addition, information specialists from the NCI-sponsored Cancer Information Service provide more than 60,000 people annually with information about prostate cancer, information about research on the disease, information about screening and treatment options, and information about coping with physical and psychological side effects of the disease and its treatment. The NCI web site provides information about prostate cancer clinical trials as well as information about treatment options for every stage of the disease.

During this summer and next fall, NCI is working with the Centers for Disease Control and Prevention and with the Health Care Financing Administration to develop an educational video for men on issues they could face about prostate cancer screening, diagnosis, and treatment. The video, intended to be relevant to a general male audience, will be developed to have special relevance to African-American men. The video will provide educational material on what men need to know about prostate cancer screening options, what they need to know about diagnostic follow if a screening test is positive, and what they need to know about treatment options if the diagnosis is positive.

NCI's basic print product about the disease, "What You Need to Know about Prostate Cancer," is now available on the web as well. It provides information about prostate cancer; its symptoms, diagnosis, staging and treatment; clinical trials; side effects of treatment; nutrition and other support for prostate cancer patients; and what prostate cancer research holds for the future.

A new publication from NCI, "Understanding Prostate Changes: A Health Guide for All Men," will soon be available on the web too. It covers all aspects of prostate cancer in more depth than the basic booklet, but also describes non-cancerous prostate conditions. Another product in development, called "Prostate Cancer Treatment: Know Your Options," will be published in print format soon and will also be available on the NCI web site.

NCI is communicating vigorously with the cancer research community. Earlier this year, NCI staff described all of the prostate cancer research initiatives that exist at the institute, and placed that information on its web site. The institute then promoted the availability of that information and issued an invitation for grant applications from the scientific community. The promotion of the information on the web site including the placement of advertisements in major scientific journals, the distribution of packets of information to the nation's cancer centers, and the distribution of information through direct mail to cancer investigators. Since the promotion began in late February, the web page listing prostate cancer grant opportunities has had thousands of hits from those seeking information about the grant opportunities.

Mr. Chairman, I appreciate the level of interest this Committee has shown in prostate cancer. I hope this plan demonstrates NIH and NCI's commitment to advancing our knowledge about prostate cancer as rapidly as possible. Our activities over the past year have invigorated the prostate cancer research community. It is this essential partnership between NIH, other funders and that research community that will successfully accomplish the ambitious goals of this plan. Dr. Varmus and I would be pleased to answer any questions you may have.

NATIONAL CANCER INSTITUTE WEB SITES

To access electronic information about prostate cancer from NCI visit our web site at: http://www.nci.nih.gov

The National Institutes of Health Report, Planning for Prostate Cancer Research will be posted: http://www.nci.nih.gov/prostateplan.html

Prostate Cancer Initiatives is available at: http://www.nci.nih.gov/prostate.html

The Prostate Cancer Progress Review Group Report is available at: http://wwwosp.nci.nih.gov/planning/prg/default.htm

OPENING STATEMENT OF SENATOR DIANNE FEINSTEIN

Senator SPECTER. We have four additional witnesses. We are going to call at this time Dr. Christopher Logothetis to join us and to present his opening round of testimony. Then we will have questions all around.

But before we do that, we have been joined by Senator Dianne Feinstein. Would you care to make an opening statement, Senator Feinstein?

Senator FEINSTEIN. Thank you very much, Mr. Chairman. I would like to put my opening statement in the record if I might.

Senator SPECTER. Without objection.

Senator FEINSTEIN. I might just say that Senator Mack and I co-chair the Senate Cancer Coalition and we have held to date six hearings on the subject of cancer. Certainly prostate cancer emerges as a major category. We found a number of problem areas that need further development. Dr. Klausner and I have been working with the American Cancer Society to try to generate a cancer dialogue, a national cancer dialogue. As a matter of fact, President Bush and Mrs. Bush are the co-chairs of that effort.

PREPARED STATEMENT

So it has been I think a very rewarding experience, and I just want to have the opportunity to welcome Dr. Klausner here, Dr. Varmus as well. I think his remarks had some good news with respect to that 63-percent increase, and I look forward to having an opportunity to ask them some questions.

So thank you, Mr. Chairman, for your leadership and for holding this hearing.

Senator SPECTER. Thank you very much, Senator Feinstein.

[The statement follows:]

PREPARED STATEMENT OF SENATOR DIANNE FEINSTEIN

Thank you, Chairman Specter for holding this hearing today on prostate cancer. The incidence of prostate cancer for all men steadily rose starting in the 1970s and then began to decline in the mid-1990s. Even with the decline, there still there will be 179,300 new cases of prostate cancer this year, including 16,300 new cases in California. There will be 37,000 deaths from prostate cancer, the second leading cause of cancer death in men.

Prostate cancer rates are highest among African American men. Mortality rates in African-American men remain more than twice as high as rates in white men.

I have heard men say, "My doctor told me if I live long enough, I will get prostate cancer." That is frightening.

RESEARCH IS KEY

As early as 2010, as our population ages, cancer incidence will increase by 29 percent. The battle against all cancers must be fought on many fronts. Congress created the National Cancer Institute in 1937. We declared the War on Cancer in 1971 and enacted a National Cancer Program. Congress has appropriated over $42 billion for cancer research since 1937. Last year, we increased the appropriation for the NCI by 13 percent, putting it now at $2.9 billion for fiscal year 1999. We increased NIH's funding by 14.6 percent. Yet sadly, we all know that we still have not done enough, when in fiscal year 1999, NCI could only fund around 30 percent of approved grants. And so, we must devote adequate funding to cancer research.

CANCER COALITION: SOME CHALLENGES

The Senate Cancer Coalition, which I co-chair with Senator Mack, has had six hearings on cancer. We have examined cancer and genetics; the promises and perils of the drug, tamoxifen; unmet challenges of breast cancer research; the implications of environmental risk factors for cancer; and new breakthroughs in cancer treatments.

In the Senate Cancer Coalition, we have been presented a number of challenges:

—*Research Funding.*—The September Cancer March's Research Task Force presented recommendations from a group of 164 leading scientists and cancer advocates, some of whom are here today, in which they called for a "national strategy to incrementally increase our investment in all areas of cancer research . . . an increase to $10 billion over the next 5 years."

—*Uneven Care.*—Experts have pointed to the April study of the Institute of Medicine which concluded that many patients do not receive care known to be effective. Describing the problem as "substantial," they say there is a big gap between what doctors would call "optimal" care and what people actually receive.

—*Clinical Trials Participation.*—Cancer March leaders stressed the need to improve clinical trials participation, testifying that only 2 (two) percent of cancer patients are enrolled in clinical trials. Of those participating, only 25 percent are elderly, even though cancer is disproportionately a disease of aging and the median age of cancer diagnosis is 68. Of people participating in clinical cancer trials, only 2–3 percent are minorities. One way of encouraging more participation, they said, is to require public and private insurers to cover routine medical costs. I am supporting a bill to do just that and will continue that push in the new Congress.

—*Expand Screening.*—We must develop effective screening methods, make sure that insurance plans cover screening for prostate and other cancers and encourage people to be screened. Congress passed prostate screening for Medicare which can save 12,000 lives a year, according to the American Foundation for Urological Disease.

—*Quality Care.*—Cancer patients have told us that they are too often disadvantaged by an uncaring—even hostile—health care climate, largely influenced by managed care plans that place arbitrary limitations on and roadblocks to care. Insurers, for example, they refuse to cover certain treatments and block access to specialists.

—*Environmental Risk Factors.*—Some experts say that insufficient attention is given to environmental risk factors that contribute to cancer's genesis and development.

—*Unexplained Patterns.*—Similarly, experts at our June 13, 1996 hearing told us that rates of many types of cancer vary between and within countries, that, for example, women in Japan have 5 times less breast cancer than women in the U.S., that rates in the northeastern U.S. are substantially higher than in the south. They said that when people migrate they tend to acquire cancer at rates closer to those of the newly adopted countries within a generation. What does this tell us? They called more research on environmental risk factors.

—*New Treatments.*—At our July 16, 1998 hearing, we heard experts outline work on several potential breakthroughs such as anti-angiogenesis, cancer vaccines, and monoclonal antibodies that hone in on specific proteins on the surface of cancer cells. They, like the September March leaders and many others, made a vigorous plea for accelerating and expanding the nation's clinical research effort, again pointing out that people over age 65 account for only 25 percent of clinical trials participants, even though the elderly are 63 percent of the National Cancer Registry.

WE NEED A BATTLE PLAN

Our nation needs a battle plan for conquering cancer. This subcommittee, by increasing funding for the National Institutes of Health has been a leading force for advancing research and today our scientists and doctors understand cancer better than efforts.

But as our witnesses will tell us today, we need to do more.

I look forward to hearing from these experts today and receiving their guidance.

OPENING STATEMENT OF SENATOR THAD COCHRAN

Senator SPECTER. Senator Cochran.

Senator COCHRAN. Thank you, Mr. Chairman. Let me just join you in welcoming these witnesses and the panel to follow. We appreciate your coming today to talk about this very important area of research. We hope that what we do in this committee assists you, helps you, supports what you are doing, and does not end up being more of a hindrance than a help.

I do mention that because I worry sometimes that we write into our legislation here and our appropriations bills some restraints or restrictions or directions that end up causing difficulties in some of the research regimes. I hope that during the course of this morning's hearing you might touch on that and give us some suggestions for restraint or in other ways guard against being an impediment to the good work that you are doing.

Senator SPECTER. Thank you, Senator Cochran.

SUMMARY STATEMENT OF CHRISTOPHER LOGOTHETIS

Senator SPECTER. Our next witness, Dr. Christopher Logothetis, is chairman of the Department of Medical Oncology at the University of Texas, the Anderson Cancer Center, also a professor; received his medical degree at the Athens School of Medicine, interned at Cook County Hospital, and is a fellow at the Anderson Cancer Senator—Center; a Freudian slip.

Dr. Logothetis, the floor is yours. Thank you.

Dr. LOGOTHETIS. Mr. Chairman and members of the subcommittee: It is a pleasure to have an opportunity to present before you. My name is Christopher Logothetis. As you mentioned, I am a professor of medicine and chairman of the Department of GU Oncology at the M.D. Anderson Cancer Center. I have had 20 years of experience treating, trying to develop therapy, and witnessing the suffering from prostate cancer. So I think I bring a unique perspective that permits me to see the changes that have occurred over time, the opportunities for the future, and to address the problems as close as one can from the eyes of the suffering.

First I would like to point out that the problem of prostate cancer is not going to go away, and it is not going to go away because our population is aging and this is an age-dependent disease. So it is going to confront us, it is going to be with us as a social, economic, and human problem.

The second thing is the baby boomers are coming into the time when they are at risk.

Third, we are the country which has the dubious distinction, as Dr. Klausner mentioned, of having the single population with the highest, most aggressive form of prostate cancer in the world. That is the African American citizens of this country. This is the worst subset of prostate cancer that exists worldwide. So it is a social, moral imperative that we simply cannot escape from.

The second dilemma that we have is who are the constituencies and how are we going to make advances? It is my belief that there are three groups that participate and will hopefully contribute to the conquest of this disease. The first groups are the patients and their families, and I think they have demonstrated in many ways, by participation in investigational trials with significant inconvenience and risk to them in trying to develop therapy—it is not uncommon in the clinic for me to hear: Even if it does not help me, I hope it will help somebody else. It is a routine statement. You would be surprised at the heroism.

The second group I think is the medical and scientific communities represented by the NCI and the NIH, the cancer centers and the universities.

The third group I think is represented by you, that is the Federal Government, to which we seek support to expand our research efforts.

What is the basis for the optimism that I think, and the opportunities for future development? I will speak from the perspective of the Cancer Center, the M.D. Anderson Cancer Center. Over the last years I have seen the disease change. When I first started treating prostate cancer I only saw patients who had widespread metastatic disease, that were immediately threatened, and that were only candidates for novel, experimental therapies. Now it is routine for me to see patients with localized disease, with many therapy options, none of which are adequate, but each of them promising and have a significant chance of altering the course.

The second thing that I have seen is I have seen the time between a laboratory or an experimental observation to the time it is confirmed as valid in the clinic and a therapy target identified be shortened dramatically. The time course for development of some new drugs that we are particularly involved with and I briefly mentioned to Dr. Klausner before, a gene therapy where we actually have identified the target gene, produced the virus, replaced the virus in humans, and seen that that virus has resulted in the production of a protein which has suppressed cancer growth in humans, has taken about 3 years. That is slow in the perspective of patients and lightning speed in the perspective of scientists and physicians.

While that is not therapy, it certainly is the basis on which we will develop therapy and represents a new foundation for treatment. Other similar examples at our institution and elsewhere exist throughout.

So how are we going to do this? Well, I think that some of the initiatives that were described by Dr. Klausner are central. NCI needs to and has demonstrated a willingness to embrace the community centers, the outreach centers, the major universities, and that is reflected in their proposal.

If you look closely at many of the studies that are being embraced by the National Cancer Institute and expanded on, they were actually developed in the cancer centers. That is not to mean that they were developed in a vacuum. They were developed with specific support from the NCI and in many ways this complements the NCI.

PREPARED STATEMENT

Finally, we need additional fundings, because if we are going to accelerate the development of therapy, if we are going to apply these quickly, if we are going to impact the illness in real time, there is nothing that replaces the resources that are required to this, and this is what we are going to have to turn to you for.

So I am optimistic and I am grateful for the opportunity, and I detect a change both in the science and clinical medicine that I believe to be very real.

Thank you.

Senator SPECTER. Thank you very much, Dr. Logothetis.

[The statement follows:]

PREPARED STATEMENT OF CHRISTOPHER J. LOGOTHETIS

Mr. Chairman and members of the Senate Subcommittee on Labor, HHS & Education Appropriations, my name is Christopher J. Logothetis. I am Professor and Chairman of the Department of Genitourinary Medical Oncology at the University of Texas—M.D. Anderson Cancer Center. I am delighted to be testifying before Senator Kay Bailey Hutchison, who represents both my cancer center and me.

I am here today on behalf of the millions of men and families whose lives have been devastated by prostate cancer. We need a national strategy to end the toll that prostate cancer takes on our nation. Simply put, Mr. Chairman, with adequate resources, prostate cancer can be prevented, controlled and cured. The NIH five-year strategy for prostate cancer research provides part of the mechanism. But it can only operate with an fiscal stream, and that means that Congress must make an appropriation of not less than $260 million for prostate cancer research at NIH in fiscal year 2000.

By most standards, prostate cancer research is underfunded. It is certainly underfunded in this country on the basis of disease burden. You already know that prostate cancer is the most commonly diagnosed nonskin cancer in America today, affecting nearly 200,000 men in 1999. You know that nearly 40,000 men will lose their lives to the disease this year. The thousands of patient visits logged each year in my clinic give testimony to the impact of prostate cancer on health care in our community, visits which are multiplied over and over at hospitals, clinics and physicians' private offices in every neighborhood and in every state. The burden of disease is particularly acute among African American men, who bear a disproportionate share of both incidence and mortality of prostate cancer.

Our population is aging, and, with the "greying" of the baby boom generation, prostate cancer will become an ever-more-important health and medical economic problem—unless changes occur now. Health economists claim that an investment in an aging population may not result in returns proportional to an investment in youth. In my opinion, prostate cancer presents a social and moral imperative that cannot be ignored. The youth of America—whose physical and emotional well being have lately been the focus of considerable national concern—need the guidance of fathers and grandfathers. Without it, they can't contribute to the welfare of this nation as they become fathers and grandfathers themselves.

Then, too, prostate cancer is not a disease that only affects older men. Fully 25 percent of cases occur in men under the age of 65, during the years that their contribution to the country is most important, economically and socially.

Prostate cancer research is also underfunded on the basis of scientific opportunity. In the past five years alone, our advancing knowledge about the biology of malignancies has shortened the time for research to get from the laboratory to the clinic. The NIH proposal makes a significant commitment to invest in this important area called "translational research."

At the same time, NIH must make a large, parallel investment in clinical research, so that new treatments can be tested thoroughly and quickly. For example, chemotherapy now works for prostate cancer, although it is not yet curative. We need to accelerate both the search for and testing of new agents to propel a cure forward.

We have also recently established that a gene can be replaced in prostate cancer cells so that proteins are produced that suppress the tumor's growth. With the appropriate investment, we can test this—and other promising therapies, like angiogenesis inhibitors, which destroy a tumor's nutrient blood supply; inhibitors of growth factors; and agents that inhibit the survival of cancer cells.

To maximize scientific opportunity, we need to assure that complementary research activities are maximized, those at NIH, at cancer centers and at university medical centers. Research successes at cancer centers and university medical centers have occurred largely because of a growing investment by NCI. We need to expand this complementary in order to rapidly test both existing therapies and novel treatments that will rapidly come "on-line."

The NIH proposal increases the number of prostate cancer SPORES, or specialized programs of research excellence. NCI has, to date, funded three prostate cancer SPORES; we need to see that network grow nationwide. SPORES—and the growth of informatics—are two crucial components of a research system that will help achieve "integration of outcomes," so that research results, particularly from clinical trials, are rapidly shared both within centers and among centers. Success will not happen in a vacuum of solitary investigation; it will happen because scientists talk to each other and aggressively share what they are learning about prostate cancer research.

The proposed additions to the QuickTrials and RAID programs will accelerate new treatments, because investigators will be able to acquire the reagents necessary for novel therapeutics and get treatments from the laboratory into the clinic. Both of these initiatives are important for the recruitment of new talent into the pool of physicians and scientists working to solve the problem of prostate cancer.

Through your leadership, Mr. Chairman, and the leadership of your colleagues, the NIH investments in prostate cancer research have jumped 60 percent from fiscal year 1998 to fiscal year 1999. We are grateful for the new talent and new opportunities that this investment—and five additional years of continued acceleration—will bring to our field. We are excited that, in addition to the potential achievements in clinical and translational research, these funding increases will see a greater number of investigator initiated research projects come to fruition. The low payline for these projects currently means that about three-quarters of worthy approved research projects—including too many in prostate cancer—go unfunded because resources aren't available.

You are now changing that. Your increasing commitment has helped prostate cancer research "get up to speed." It is now time to give research the resources to win the race. Cure is possible. You can help make it happen. The men and families whose lives have been touched by this horrible disease know that you must make it happen.

Thank you, Mr. Chairman.

OPENING STATEMENT OF SENATOR TED STEVENS

Senator SPECTER. I am told that we have an extraordinarily long line outside and I am wondering if we might not be able to bring some more people in in the corners, and we could even have some people sitting in the Senators' chairs until the Senators arrive, so that we can try to admit as many people as we can to the hearing room.

We have been joined by our distinguished chairman of the full committee, who has some special insights on this subject. Senator Stevens, would you care to make an opening statement?

Senator STEVENS. Well, I would ask you to put my statement in the record in view of the fact that I am late.

Senator SPECTER. Without objection.

Senator STEVENS. My insight is that I am a fellow survivor along with Senator Dole and Mr. Milken, Mike, and others, and I am very interested to see that you are pursuing this to the depth you are, Mr. Chairman. So I congratulate you and look forward to the statements.

Doctor, nice to see you.

[The statement follows:]

PREPARED STATEMENT OF SENATOR TED STEVENS

Mr. Chairman, I'm pleased that you are holding this hearing today to hear from NIH about the report which our Committee requested them to develop to highlight the steps that NIH is taking to enhance its prostate cancer research program. I am looking forward to hearing from Dr. Varmus and Dr. Klausner.

I also welcome my friends former Senate Majority Leader Bob Dole and Mike Milken—and Mr. Joe Torre of the New York Yankees. We are all part of the fraternity of prostate cancer survivors—and we are all exerting our best efforts to help find a cure and more effective treatments for this disease which continues to be the most frequently occurring cancer (aside from skin cancer), representing 29 percent of all new cancer cases in American men, and costing as much as $15 billion per year, including medical care and lost wages and productivity.

Just last week, the Senate passed the Department of Defense Appropriations bill for fiscal year 2000, which contains $100 million in funding for research on prostate cancer. But, as I continue to remind my friends in the prostate cancer advocacy groups, I believe that our main focus for medical research, including funds for prostate cancer, must continue to be in the National Institutes of Health. I believe strongly that we must continue to fund medical research at a level which will allow us to take advantage of rapidly developing biotechnology breakthroughs in finding causes, cures and treatments for diseases like prostate cancer. I look forward to hearing NIH's blueprint for prostate cancer research that will lead us forward toward a cure and better treatment.

PSA TESTING

Senator SPECTER. We will begin now the 5-minute round of questions by Senators, and I shall begin.

Dr. Klausner, I think it will be useful if you would describe what the PSA test is, what men need to know about it, and to comment about its accuracy in detecting prostate cancer.

Dr. KLAUSNER. Yes. The PSA test is a blood test that detects a protein that is pretty uniquely produced by prostate cells, not prostate cancer cells, but either prostate cancer cells or normal prostate cells, that leaks into the blood with the structural changes in the prostate of often relatively early prostate cancer.

It is absolutely clear that PSA is capable of detecting prostate cancer, and in fact the dramatic change in the profile, the distribution of newly diagnosed prostate cancer from late disease to early disease, is overwhelmingly due to the introduction and the widespread use of this test.

Senator SPECTER. How reliable is it?

Dr. KLAUSNER. Well, PSA itself does not mean prostate cancer is present. If the PSA is elevated beyond a certain level, and especially if its rate of rise is followed, it is an alarm that says there may be prostate cancer there. There are other things that may cause a rise in PSA.

Senator SPECTER. If PSA does not sound the alarm, does that still mean the individual might have prostate cancer?

Dr. KLAUSNER. Individuals may have very microscopic prostate cancer or very well differentiated and localized prostate cancer that has not led to the structural changes in the prostate and still have normal PSA. But PSA is a very good test for detecting prostate cancer.

Senator SPECTER. Dr. Varmus, what would the funding have to be for the National Cancer Institute, NIH, so that you granted research funds for all the meritorious applications?

Dr. VARMUS. It is a difficult question, Senator, because we cannot anticipate exactly how many applications we will have in the future. As you know, we currently award funds to roughly 30 to 35 percent of our applicants. We view the vast majority of the applications we receive as meritorious at some level—that is, worthy of support if resources were totally unlimited.

We recognize that the Federal Government does not have totally unlimited resources; therefore, we use peer review to stratify those applications.

Senator SPECTER. The allocation of the resources is up to the Congress, and I believe we have very extensive resources. As I said earlier, $1.7 trillion. We are a very rich country and I believe Americans would be prepared to pay whatever it took. So we need to know from you what the NIH budget should be, what the National Cancer Institute budget should be, so that all the meritorious applications may be granted.

I know your figures went up from the high twenties into the low to mid thirties when we increased your funding.

Dr. VARMUS. That is correct.

Senator SPECTER. But the next line of questioning is, what would it take to fund all of the meritorious application? Would you give that some thought and report back to the committee?

Dr. VARMUS. We can also tell you that in the report we have submitted there is a professional judgment budget that gives some notion of what we think we would need to pursue most or all of the goals that we think are meritorious. This is not to fund all the applications, but to pursue those meritorious goals. The numbers are provided in the report.

Senator SPECTER. OK, we will review that and see if we have a follow-up question.

Dr. VARMUS. Thank you.

Senator SPECTER. Dr. Logothetis, you comment, and understandably so, about prostate cancer being a part of the aging process. In these hearings we are always asking perhaps the impossible question about a cure for cancer. We have had some hearings on stem cells recently and on Parkinson's disease. We have heard estimates that perhaps 5 years, 10 years at the outside, Parkinson's disease may be cured.

I would like your evaluation as to the possibility of curing—I know when you talk about cancer there are many different forms. But what is the possibility, theoretical, of curing cancer? What is the possibility of curing prostate cancer?

Dr. LOGOTHETIS. I guess the best statement is it is hard until it is easy. I think that there is a view on how we can get there that has a reasonable chance of significantly altering the course of this illness and can lead to cure. Let me describe how I think that that will happen.

First of all, I do not think that there is a single drug that will develop that will cure this disease. It has not happened in the other curable diseases. There will have to be a convergence of events that will cure the disease. One is we will have to detect the disease earlier. My optimism comes from the fact that that has already happened. As mentioned, I rarely see advanced disease.

Second is we will have to make technological advances in the imaging of the prostate so we can actually deliver drugs to the prostate very easy and monitor its effectiveness in a functional way.

Third, we are going to have to change our views of how we intervene and how we sort of view this disease. Let me describe. The traditional approach to prostate cancer is that it is not a disease until it is cancer. If a general internist who is taking care of heart disease waited until you had a heart attack to intervene, that would be considered irrational.

What we view this as is a chronic degenerative disease that has a process that precedes its malignant manifestation—high blood pressure followed by a heart attack—and we are waiting until the late event, and we are actually only treating the late event and then not intervening with the processes that are contributing.

I think that once that cultural change has occurred, which I already see has changed, early intervention happens. We will have a strategy including new drugs, new technology, and a willingness of the population to be treated that has a chance of curing this disease, between 5 and 10 years would be my guess if you were to ask. Now, I am cured an incurable optimist, so I have a form of cancer, too. But I think it is real, and you can see it when you look at patients and see the changes over time.

Senator SPECTER. Thank you very much.

My time has expired. Under our early bird rule, we turn now to Senator Feinstein.

Senator FEINSTEIN. Thank you very much, Mr. Chairman.

Perhaps, Dr. Logothetis, I should ask you this question. Dr. Peter Rosen, a UCLA professor and co-director of UCLA's Advanced Prostate Cancer Clinic, is quoted in UCLA Medicine by saying this: "The last important discovery that impacted the treatment of prostate cancer was made in the 1940's." Do you agree with that?

Dr. LOGOTHETIS. No. The last important one that has been applied, it is correct. We have spent from the forties until very recently, a long period of time, suppressing the growth of prostate cancer by suppressing male hormone production. It is true that there has not been a wide application of the new moves and I think that there is ample evidence that PSA has changed the disease in how it presents to us and has changed the clinical problem.

So while I agree that there has not been a fundamental applied change in the disease that has spread, I disagree that there have not been significant advances in the disease.

Senator FEINSTEIN. Now, on page two of your remarks you say that chemotherapy now works for prostate cancer, although it is not yet curative.

Dr. LOGOTHETIS. Yes.

Senator FEINSTEIN. And just a few moments ago you mentioned that there probably has to be, at least I thought you said, some interrelationship between drugs that we do not yet know about. Is that interrelationship between drugs or other techniques, like radioactivity or radiation?

Dr. LOGOTHETIS. Let me maybe place the question in a perspective. In order to prove cure in prostate cancer, it would take 10 years for us to detect a difference. But the degree of effectiveness of the combination chemotherapies which are currently being used and are now widely applied has reached a level where it is equal to that seen in other common solid tumors, such as breast cancer, such as some forms of lung cancer, where it impacts survival.

What is missing is the piece of giving chemotherapy early to see if it affects survival.

Senator FEINSTEIN. That is where screening comes in.

Dr. LOGOTHETIS. It is screening to detect it early and apply therapy, which clearly helps patients with advanced disease, clearly helps them, in a setting, as Dr. Klausner said, where we can now exploit the advantage that we have been furnished with by PSA detection by treating patients earlier and then applying the biological techniques to select the proper patient for such therapy.

I think that those events are converging.

Senator FEINSTEIN. Interesting.

Now, I did not know that the United States has the most virulent form of prostate cancer in the world. Why would that be and what would the genesis of that be?

Dr. LOGOTHETIS. Again, we have the most virulent form in our African American citizens, and that is important because obviously they suffer and die more from the disease. But it is also very important because it provides a tremendous amount of insight into the events that may lead to this disease that may have wider application.

We do not know the specific mechanisms. It is reasonable to implicate diet. It is reasonable to implicate all sorts of environmental factors. It is probably genetically not so uniform. It is a heterogeneous population, more heterogeneous, more different than one would think. But if you were to ask me to guess, it is going to be social and dietary factors that are more likely to be implicated in this.

Senator FEINSTEIN. Dr. Klausner, Dr. Varmus, can you add to that?

Dr. KLAUSNER. Well, I think Dr. Logothetis is right, it is most likely to be exogenous factors, although again across the populations there are some different distributions of inherited common variations, for example in the androgen receptor gene, in the vitamin D receptor gene. So there may be some biologic differences. It is true African Americans are a diverse population. But there are differences generally in the population between Asians, Caucasians, and African Americans, in the distribution of certain biological characteristics that may also have an effect.

But I suspect, as most of us do, that it is probably due to dietary or environmental factors. But we do not know, though we have been looking, what those dietary factors are.

Dr. VARMUS. It is perhaps useful to distinguish between the incidence and the mortality of the disease. There is about 30 percent higher incidence of prostate cancer among African Americans than among Caucasians in our country, and about a twofold increase in the death rate.

We think that most of that disparity in death rate is due to the speed with which people seek care and perhaps the level of care. In studies that the National Cancer Institute has carried out using a control between African American and white patients, African Americans seem to respond equally well to the therapies that have been tested. So it is not clear that the response is different to the therapies that are being developed.

The issue with respect to genetics is an important one. Investigators at the National Human Genome Research Institute have identified at least two chromosomal sites at which there is a gene predisposing individuals to prostate cancer. However, we have no evidence as yet that those genes are more likely to be mutated in African American populations.

Senator FEINSTEIN. I see the red light. Thank you, Mr. Chairman. Thank you very much.

Senator SPECTER. Thank you very much, Senator Feinstein.

Senator Cochran.

Senator COCHRAN. Mr. Chairman, thank you.

In Dr. Logothetis' testimony you mentioned the fact that prostate cancer research is underfunded on the basis of scientific opportunity. This goes to the question I think the chairman asked Dr. Varmus earlier. You then say: "The NIH proposal makes a significant commitment to invest in an important area called translational research." What is that and how does that offer promise for dealing with this disease?

Dr. LOGOTHETIS. One of the challenges in medical research and in cancer research specifically is to bridge the gap between exciting observations in the laboratory and their application in the clinic. The whole processes that make up that difference, that big canyon, is translational research. It requires the sort of methodical, plodding type of research that frequently is not exciting, to get all the information from large populations, target the subset with your appropriate therapy.

So I would call translational research the process by which one prioritizes, learns, and finally applies successfully therapy based on exciting ideas that have been developed in the clinic. That is a big, big chasm.

Senator COCHRAN. Would it be helpful—and I am directing this at Dr. Varmus and Dr. Klausner—to earmark funds for this purpose or are you more comfortable with a more general provision of just money and letting you decide based on the applications you get for the research? Do we make a mistake by earmarking for something specific like this?

Dr. VARMUS. We favor some position in between, Senator. As you know, there are many problems that we believe could be pursued more vigorously with more funds, prostate cancer and many others. We are a public institution. We are responsive to the concerns of the public, manifested in the Congress, and we do want to know what concerns you and the public most.

It obviously makes life more difficult for us to have to shape the research agenda to fit a specific dollar assignation. We hope that we can illustrate this principle today in the conduct of prostate cancer research, as well as in the context of other diseases, by showing you how effectively and speedily we can respond to that clear public concern, and indeed the increased incidence and severity of the disease, by shaping a research program that does reflect a deeper commitment than is evident from the overall increase in funding of the NIH.

Senator COCHRAN. Another specific undertaking—and I think this is in the statement of Dr. Klausner—the Environmental Genome Project. Tell us about that? Should we try to target funds for that as well?

Dr. KLAUSNER. The Environmental Genome Project is a project of the National Institute of Environmental Health Sciences. It is an attempt to identify common variations in genes across the human population. We recognize that the future of medicine in many ways will be driven by understanding why one person is different from another. There are dramatic examples of that. If you have two people who smoke, one person gets cancer, the other does not, why? And on and on. How they respond to therapy, etcetera.

We all believe that this in part relates to the millions of variations between any two individuals that are not identical twins. So that project actually dovetails with many projects across the NIH, including one NCI released just last week, where we are annotating genes in a database for all researchers to use that lay out the common variations. These variations will be essential in interpreting research, clinical trials, and environmental studies.

In fact, we think one of the reasons it has been so difficult to pinpoint environmental causes is because it is not the environment per se, but it is the interaction of the environment, the complexity of the environment, with individual variations, how they metabolize things, how they respond.

So this is going to be the new world of applying this approach of variation genetics to all aspects of our research, and the project that you are talking about is one of the integrated set of projects that all of the Institutes are involved in to get that information and to make it available to the research community.

Senator COCHRAN. Thank you, Mr. Chairman.

Senator SPECTER. Thank you very much, Senator Cochran.

Senator Stevens.

Senator STEVENS. I have got real trouble with the way the NIH has been handling prostate cancer. It has led to an increased demand on our defense appropriations bill and a different approach in the Department of Defense to the allocation of the money that we provide from that bill for prostate cancer research.

Despite the fact that there has been a substantial increase in the last 20 years in prostate cancer incidence, or detection, whichever you want to say, you have had practically a flat line in terms of prostate cancer research coming out of NIH.

Can you tell me, why is that?

Dr. KLAUSNER. Well, I think it has not been a flat line. I can describe what we have done for the last 4 years since I have been there. In each year we have increased the amount of prostate cancer research spending, actually for each of the 4 years, out of proportion to the growth of the budget, with this year's 63 percent increase compared to the 15 percent increase that we have had.

But more important than the numbers—the numbers are important, and we have talked about this with this committee before— there are in prostate cancer and in fact as far as I can see in all of our cancer research more possibilities, more needs than we have resources for. So our approach has been both to increase the funding, which we have done and we think quite significantly, as well as to make sure that that is coupled with the most effective and efficient way to spend, which involves setting priorities, bringing the broad communities together to tell us, not for us to tell them, what those priorities ought to be, by developing a real, for us for the first time, prostate cancer research plan, which we initiated almost as soon as I began, and to coordinate the activities between NCI and other funders of prostate cancer research, whether it is the Department of Defense or private funders, which we have moved to do, so that whatever dollars are there, inadequate to the task for this cancer and others, we make the best use of them.

Senator STEVENS. As a matter of fact, I am more and more of the opinion that we should follow the matching fund concept and put all Federal dollars into a pot and say we will match, we will provide 25 percent or whatever it might be of the funding necessary for the projects that the private sector will put its money into, and stop some of the costs that are associated with the way you handle money.

You have built two brand new buildings out there in the time that we have been trying to increase prostate cancer research. As a matter of fact, the last time I went out to that campus I did not even recognize it. I hope you will do me the honor not to name a building after me, because my predecessors all have buildings out there now, and I really do not think that is what you should be into.

You should be finding a way to handle this money so the public gets the best return for the dollars we are spending from the taxpayers' money.

PROSTATE CANCER IN MINORITY POPULATIONS

Incidentally, the statistics—and no offense to the black people who are here—the highest incidence of cancer in the United States is in the indigenous people. You somehow or other separate the Alaska Native people from the American Indian people and as a consequence got two categories. If you add them up, the indigenous people of the United States have the highest cancer incidence. I do not think we have ever explored that, have we? Why is it that we sort of overlook that? But American Indians and Alaska Natives, add them together, they have the highest cancer incidence and they have the highest number of deaths.

Have you ever explored that? Why?

Dr. KLAUSNER. Yes. In fact, the reason we know that number is because NCI has a surveillance system, called SEER, to monitor the rates in Alaska among a variety of Native American populations, and then whenever we see changes in patterns, we provide funding to do special studies, which we are doing in Alaska and elsewhere, to try to understand why patterns are different.

Prostate cancer rates are relatively low in both of those populations, although the survival rates are very poor compared to virtually all other groups with cancer. But the incidence rates in fact are, for prostate cancer, much lower in Native Americans and Alaska Natives than in the white, Hispanic, or African American community.

ADMINISTRATIVE COSTS RELATED TO RESEARCH

Senator STEVENS. I have got one last question. What is your overhead cost? When we put up $10 million for cancer research, how much actually goes out the door to someone doing the research?

Dr. KLAUSNER. Yes. Our administrative cost for running the Institute is approximately 4 percent of the total budget.

Senator STEVENS. That is not what I asked. What are you holding back from when I put up $10 million? How much goes out the door to contracts?

Dr. KLAUSNER. Well, about 15 percent of our budget is spent on research at the campus. We have a big intramural research program, and that is research. I assume you are talking about what gets spent in research. Essentially, everything but the administrative cost, which is about 4 percent, gets spent on research. Eighty-five percent leaves Bethesda, goes throughout the country to support cancer centers and projects everywhere, and about 15 percent is for intramural. Then we divide the administrative cost, which is about 4 percent, across those.

Senator STEVENS. Where does that tremendous construction cost fit into that, doctor?

Dr. VARMUS. The construction costs, Senator, are in our B and F budget for the intramural program. I should emphasize the nature of the buildings that you are seeing. First of all, one building is being constructed to replace laboratory buildings that were constructed in the 1940's, which are unsafe by the criteria of many evaluations for current laboratory work. Another building is to replace the clinical research building, in which all our clinical research activity is carried out, which was constructed in 1953, and which was again recommended for replacement or demolition by the Army Corps of Engineers and many others. And the third is a small building that is being constructed to support our important new vaccine research initiative directed against HIV and other novel infectious agents.

Overall, the NIH spends, as Dr. Klausner indicated, between 3 and 4 percent of its budget on administrative costs. When our money is sent to extramural institutions, on the average about one-third of the dollars are spent at those institutions for facilities and administrative costs and the rest for direct application to research.

Senator STEVENS. I am going to pursue that later.

Thank you very much.

Senator SPECTER. Thank you, Senator Stevens.

Thank you very much, Dr. Logothetis, Dr. Klausner, and Dr. Varmus. We very much appreciate your testimony.

I would like to turn now to Senator Dole, Mr. Milken, and Mr. Torre. Our first witness is the distinguished former majority leader of the United States Senate, Senator Bob Dole. Senator Dole began his public career by playing end on the Russell High School football team in 1941, was a basketball star, and as late as 1996 Dr. Erwin Luthey, the coach of the debate team, noted his absence from the State championship debate team in 1941 in Russell, Kansas.

Senator Dole served in——

Senator STEVENS. Pardon me. Is there not sort of an emphasis on Russell, Kansas? What is that for?

Senator SPECTER. To draw your attention, Senator Stevens.

Senator DOLE. Appropriations, you know, money.

Senator STEVENS. That the two of you are each from Russell, Kansas, yes, OK.

Senator SPECTER. This is all in the staff's introductory comments, Senator Stevens. I always read it verbatim.

He served in the Kansas legislature, was county attorney in Russell. Interesting story: was drafted by both political parties, checked the registration, and accepted the Republican nomination, was county attorney.

Served four terms in the House of Representatives from 1960, to election to the Senate in 1968; the chairman of the National Republican Party, vice presidential Republican nominee in 1976, presidential nominee in 1996, and star witness today, and who knows for the future.

Senator Dole, the floor is yours.

SUMMARY STATEMENT OF HON. BOB DOLE

Senator DOLE. Thank you very much for that very kind introduction, which I sent up to you, and I appreciate your repeating it. [Laughter.]

I saw Stevens rolling in this morning in a convertible. You looked good in there, Ted, so that is great.

But I am very honored to be here with two very distinguished gentlemen in this case: Michael Milken, who we all know has been sort of pioneering efforts with real money and all the things that it takes, and traveling all over the country and all over the world, and I applaud his efforts; and then Joe Torre. I have always been a Yankee fan, Joe.

Mr. TORRE. I was not always a Yankee fan.

Senator DOLE. I go back to DiMaggio and Gehrig and those days, when I knew all the earned run averages and how many two-base hits, triples. I had them all memorized. It has been some time ago. Joe is a recent, well, survivor.

I want to thank all the men and their wives, spouses, who may be here also. I would just summarize my statement, because I think we are here to underscore the importance of research and also the importance of reaching out for new technologies.

I had this all happen to me 8 years ago and it happened to Ted just a little before then. I would say there is no doubt about it, the reason we have had an increase in research funds has been largely due to Senator Stevens' efforts. I remember getting a very—when I said we are going to increase prostate cancer research, I got a very nasty letter from a constituent. It said: There you go helping yourself again.

Well, it was too late for me. I mean, it was already gone. I was thinking more about her son or her grandson, and I think many of these survivors who are here today have that same feeling.

One thing that we do that maybe others do on the committee, we have a Bob Dole Screening Booth at the Kansas State Fair and we do mammograms and PSA's. We have been doing it for, I do not know, 8, 10 years. One thing I discovered, I finally figured it out. When I was no longer the Majority Leader, the funding dropped a little from the drug companies, so it is a little harder to raise the money now for the PSA tests and the mammograms. But I think it is an excellent idea, and we probably find we do about 3 or 4,000 and probably, I do not know how many, a hundred or so men discover they have a prostate problem they did not know about.

So I will use this opportunity today to say again, if you are a male over age 40, particularly if you have a family history, ask your doctor about getting a prostate checkup.

People ask me how I can be so open about my own experience with prostate cancer, and I must admit that I decided to go public before the operation because I think silence can be deadly. Almost by default, I have become some sort of a spokesperson for prostate cancer. I have talked to hundreds of men across the country and their wives. In fact, yesterday I talked to the Mayor of Wichita, Kansas, who is having surgery tomorrow morning, to reassure him that it was going to be fine.

But I must say I think the media needs to be educated on not only what happens, but side effects and all the other things, because I can tell you some are very, very insensitive to a real, real problem that affects the man and the spouse, and hopefully that is a matter of education.

There are all kinds of treatments out there. Senator Helms had radiation. We had surgery. I think my first awareness of prostate cancer and how serious it was was on the death of my good friend Spark Matsunaga, who suffered and suffered and suffered with prostate cancer and it spread and it spread. I do not know which—you can have radiation, you can have surgery. I do not know which is the best. I had surgery and 8 years later my PSA is negligible, so I assume I made the right decision.

But it has been indicated here this morning by the three experts there are all these other things happening out there looking for new treatment options. I think one of these days it will be a thing of the past. He said 5 to 10 years, and I think maybe Michael may comment on that, too.

But I think it is an important thing for us to think about, whether we are prepared to take the steps that are necessary so when we have this new technology for treatment becomes available we are going to have access to it. You have got to have access or it is not going to be much good.

Let me just quickly; I see the red light snapping there. One example is the proposed change in the reimbursement rate for an innovative prostate cancer treatment known as brachytherapy. This therapy involves the implantation of radioactive seeds in the prostate directly. You go in and do it in the afternoon, you are in the swimming pool the next day. I do not know how—they still do not have enough experience how effective it is, but these seeds emit radiation that destroys cancer cells while minimizing exposure for surrounding tissues. For some patients this very minimal procedure, done on an outpatient basis, can treat some forms of cancer.

Now, currently Medicare reimburses for this procedure, but if the reimbursement is reduced as proposed right now this type of technology is going to be gone.

I would say in the interest of full disclosure I also serve on an advisory board of a California company called Endocare, and they do this cryosurgery. They freeze the prostate. Again, that is making about a half-inch incision. They freeze the prostate and you go home. It is all in an afternoon.

Now, as Senator Stevens and others know who have had prostate surgery, that takes a while. In addition to the hospitalization, it takes 6 to 8 weeks or more to regain your strength.

So I say there are new technologies there. There are things happening. And one of these days it is going to be at least, if not cured, at least other options for patients. So I just commend this committee. We are talking about the baby boomers and 77 million of these in the year 2011. The demand is going to be high. There is going to be more pressure for funds from this committee and other committees. Of course, by the year—I would ask that my statement be made part of the record——

Senator SPECTER. Without objection.

PREPARED STATEMENT

Senator DOLE [continuing]. And just close by saying in the year 2011 Michael Milken and CapCURE will have found a cure for prostate cancer, Joe Torre will own the Yankees——

Mr. TORRE. No, thanks.

Senator DOLE [continuing]. And I will be writing my memoirs on being the country's First Gentleman.

Thank you very much.

Senator SPECTER. Thank you very much, Senator Dole. As usual, thank you.

[The statement follows:]

PREPARED STATEMENT OF SENATOR BOB DOLE

Mr. Chairman, Senator Harkin: Thank you for inviting me here this morning to discuss prostate cancer. It seems that just about every family in America has been touched in some way by cancer. My family has. And, I have.

Over eight years ago I was diagnosed with prostate cancer. I was lucky to have had the disease diagnosed early and treated promptly through surgery.

Eight years later, I am happy to say I am cancer free. Since the time of my diagnosis I have tried to speak out as much as possible about the value and importance of early detection. I truly believed then, and continue to believe today, that early detection saved my life. The cancer was found when it was still contained within the prostate gland and when I had a variety of treatment options from which to choose.

I will use this opportunity today to say it again: If you're a male over age 40, particularly if you have a family history, ask your doctor about getting a prostate check up. People ask me how I can be so open about my own experience with prostate cancer. I must admit, when I first started speaking out about this disease there were plenty of awkward moments. But, then I decided that the alternative—silence—can be deadly.

So, when I am fortunate enough to be asked to testify before Congress on this issue, I do it.

While my message of the importance of early detection is one that I will continue to deliver, I would like to take a moment to talk about treatment options.

When I was diagnosed, I was basically given two options: Surgery or radiation. That was it. I was told of the side effects of both, the risks of the procedures, and the probability for cure. I have to admit, it was almost a toss up. Both had side effects that sounded unpleasant, to say the least, but both also had high rates of success. I chose surgery. And, since I am cancer free today, I of course believe I made the right decision.

But, every day there is a scientist looking for the cure for cancer, or looking for a new treatment option. And, one of these days—I think in the not so distant future—there will be a cure. But, the question is will we recognize it when we see it? And, I think that is an important question for Members of Congress and the administration to think about. Is our Government prepared to take the steps that are necessary so that when a new technology for treatment becomes available, patients with the disease can access it?

One example is a proposed change in the reimbursement rate for an innovative prostate treatment known as brachytherapy. This therapy involves the implantation of radioactive seeds into the prostate directly. The seeds emit radiation that destroy cancer cells while minimizing exposure to surrounding tissues. For some patients, this minimally invasive procedure, done on an outpatient basis, has been shown to treat some forms of prostate cancer.

Currently, Medicare reimburses for this procedure. But, if the reimbursement is reduced, as is currently proposed, this type of technology will become less available to patients.

I am on the advisory board of a company that makes a cryosurgical device that freezes the prostate so that the cancer can no longer grow. When I had my surgery, I was in the hospital for a week and recovering for months. With cryosurgery, a patient can leave the hospital the same day and return to work the next.

It's not for every patient, of course, but neither is surgery. Yet, despite it's success, Medicare took three years to cover this procedure, and it actually will not begin coverage until next month. I wonder how many patients could have benefited from cryosurgery, but couldn't because of the Government's reimbursement policies.

Please do not misunderstand me. I have been and will continue to be an advocate for Medicare's solvency. But, as our health care system continues to evolve and change, policy makers must encourage the adoption of innovative therapies. What's the point of science making advances everyday if there is no way to deliver the technologies to patients who need them?

The private sector readily accepts new therapies partly because they are often cost effective, but mostly because the consumers in the market demand them. As the baby boomers age, I believe Medicare will feel the same pressure from its consumers.

When the country's 77 million baby boomers start becoming Medicare eligible in 2011, the Government is going to have to deliver—the demand will be so high. In order to satisfy that demand, the Medicare Program will have to be modernized. That means looking at new therapies and keeping pace with scientific advances.

Of course, in 2011, Michael Milken and CapCURE will have found a cure for prostate cancer, Joe Torre will own the Yankees, and I will be writing my memoirs on being the country's "first gentleman".

Thank you very much.

SUMMARY STATEMENT OF MICHAEL MILKEN

Senator SPECTER. We turn now to our next witness. This panel happens to be in alphabetical order. Michael Milken, founder and Chairman of CapCURE, the Association for the Cure of Cancer of the Prostate. Mr. Milken is a cancer survivor, having been diagnosed with prostate cancer in February of 1993, a graduate of the University of California at Berkeley, a Master's from the Wharton School at the University of Pennsylvania.

Thank you for all you are doing, Mr. Milken. We look forward to your testimony.

Mr. MILKEN. Thank you, Mr. Chairman and members of the subcommittee. It is a pleasure to be here today.

Not only am a 6-year survivor of prostate cancer, I have lost 10 of my closest relatives to various forms of cancer in the last few years.

I think I would like to just touch on today three or four items. One of them particularly is investment. I do not believe the American public is fully aware of the amount of money that our country has invested in cancer research since the war was declared in 1971. This year we will spend less than four thousandths of one percent of the GDP on cancer research and we will spend less than 20 cents on a dollar—out of $100 that we have in the Federal budget, less than 20 cents goes to cancer research. In spite of the fact that one in two men and one in three women will get cancer, we are investing less than 20 cents out of $100.

This is one of the few areas in the world where you spend 30 to 40 times as much money on care as on research in trying to solve the problem. There is no private industry, there is no private company, that could afford to continue in business spending 30 to 40 times as much money on servicing the problem and care as to do on correcting the problem. It makes no sense for private industry and it makes no sense for government.

The Federal Government has made extraordinary investments long term in our country's infrastructure. The interstate highway system is a case in point. We believe it is now time to make a similar investment in our country's human capital, which holds the great values for the next century. The suffering of cancer patients and the grief of families and friends are beyond calculation.

But some distinguished economists, including Kevin Murphy, who recently won the award as the world's greatest economist under 40, have attempted to calculate the economic value to our country of cancer. Based on his calculations, the 560,000 Americans who will die this year alone from cancer will result in a loss of value to the United States measured in trillions, not billions, of dollars.

The 560,000 fathers, mothers, brothers, sisters, neighbors, and friends, that is approximately the same number of men and women who served in Desert Storm. Imagine the reaction of the country if General Schwartzkopf had announced that no Americans sent to the Gulf were coming home, not one had survived. Imagine that impact. That happens every year in America.

Opportunity costs. The approximately $2.9 billion that the Federal Government will invest in cancer research allows the NCI to fund, as we have heard, approximately 30 percent of approved grants. But this is just the tip of the iceberg. As many of our country's leading young scientists have told us, many of them have been told if they go into cancer research, particularly prostate cancer research, it is professional suicide. There is not enough money available. If they choose that for their career, they will be little known in the future.

In addition to that, when they see Nobel Prize winners' and others programs not funded that have been approved, they see little hope and opportunity for themselves in this career. We discourage our best and brightest to go into the field of prostate cancer research and cancer research, rather than encourage them.

When the war was declared on cancer in 1971 and promise of a solution in a decade, the same as President Kennedy's earlier goal of putting a man on the moon, which was achieved in less than 10 years, many thought it would work, and many of the news services recently have pointed out that people expected us to have a cure for cancer, not put a man on the moon by the end of this century.

We thought this because when President Roosevelt declared a war on polio it produced a Salk vaccine. My family knows something about polio because my father contracted it as a child, and I was among the first of the baby boomers to receive that vaccine. A very simple concept: Get a shot, wipe out a disease. Surely we should be able to do the same for cancer.

At The National Cancer Summit in 1995, General Schwartzkopf pointed out for military lessons—we can apply this to the war on cancer—there comes a time when, he said, we must get on with the battle. You never have perfect intelligence on the enemy. The fact is we have plenty of information for the offensive. We lack sufficient firepower.

How much firepower do we need? On September 25, 1998, when 600 organizations came here to testify and participate in the march in front of Senators Mack and Feinstein, I suggested we needed at least $10 billion a year for cancer research, at least $10 billion. That is $40 per American. It is a fraction of the cost of failure, of treating more than 100 million Americans who are currently living who are expected to get cancer in their lifetime. A $100 investment for each American who is expected to get cancer today might save us $100,000 in expenditures per American later.

It is embarrassing when we see single companies invest more money in their own R&D and capital expenditures than our entire Federal Government spends on cancer research. One, and not the largest investor, Intel Corporation, spends more than twice as much money on their R&D and capital expenditures as the Federal Government spends on cancer research.

Senator SPECTER. Mr. Milken, I am sorry to interrupt you. They have just called a vote and we can come back later. Are you available to wait a few minutes? There are two votes. If we go at the very end of the first vote and pick up the second vote, we will not be gone too long. But I know you are all busy men.

Senator DOLE. The Yankees won last night, so he feels——

Mr. TORRE. I am safe for a couple hours, anyway.

Mr. MILKEN. I do not think we can think of anything that is more important, Senator.

Senator SPECTER. If you can return, I would like to explore when we finish the rounds of questioning how we can stimulate more public concern and more funding, which is really what we need to do. So if you can wait, we will not rush Mr. Milken.

Proceed.

Mr. MILKEN. I will just make a couple brief points here. Education has been the subject of many of our leaders, and one of our great education leaders said: "If you think education is expensive, try ignorance." I think if you think of investment in cancer research as expensive, try paying for the treatment of 100 million Americans who are going to get cancer.

I would like to make two more points, and some of them are beyond the scope of this committee. I believe that Congress and the Senate should consider a tax incentive for research such as enhanced investment tax credits. If we could do it for automobiles, maybe we could also do it for cancer. The ability to sell tax loss carryforward for the biotech companies of our country, who lost $2.5 billion last year, investing $7.5 billion in R&D—if we have a real war on cancer, why do we not issue cancer war bonds? I would be happy to buy $50 million of them myself.

Why not extend patent lives, accelerate FDA approvals, and authorize direct contracting of corporations for R&D? It is the kind of public-private partnership that helped us win World War Two and could help us win the war on cancer.

I believe in all these proposals that we can accelerate science. If we give cancer researchers the same kind of tools that the cancer companies see out there in technology companies and employ them for scientific development, we can move things along faster.

PREPARED STATEMENT

It is up to you, Mr. Chairman, and your colleagues to provide and direct the necessary resources to pave the way. We owe this not to ourselves, but to our families and future generations. You have strived to leave our children and Nation free of debt and a world free from war, a world that cherishes the sanctity of a single human life. Yet we have lost 11 million Americans to the war on cancer since it was declared and we have not been willing to make the investment to find a solution to this problem. This is a sad legacy for those of us in the baby boomer generation to leave to our children.

We need your help. We welcome your support. Thank you very much.

Senator SPECTER. Thank you very much, Mr. Milken.

[The statement follows:]

PREPARED STATEMENT OF MICHAEL MILKEN

Mr. Chairman and members of the Subcommittee on Labor, Health & Human Services and Education Appropriations, my name is Michael Milken. I am Founder, President and Chairman of CaP CURE, the Association for the Cure of Cancer of the Prostate—the world's largest private funder of prostate cancer research. I am a six-year survivor of prostate cancer, and I have lost 10 close relatives to cancer.

The federal investment in finding cures for cancer—$3 billion annually—is less than zero point zero zero zero four percent of our gross domestic product, or about one-seventh of what Americans spend on beauty products. At the same time, we often hear that our nation is spending more than $100 billion annually—much of it by the federal government—for cancer care. With the graying of the baby- boom generation and its greater risk of cancer as members pass the age of 50, cancer-care dollars are likely to double within a decade. Is there any organization that would spend more than 35 times as much money to deal with the effects of a problem as it would to solve the problem? It makes no sense in the private sector, and, with current concerns about spending rates and budget caps, it should make no sense in government.

The federal government has, for example, made extraordinary investments—long-term—in components of the country's infrastructure; the interstate highway system is a case in point. It is now time to make a similar commitment in human capital. The suffering of cancer patients and the grief of their families and friends are beyond calculation. But some distinguished economists—such as Kevin Murphy at the University of Chicago—have calculated the economic value of the lives lost. These figures amplify cancer's already staggering annual morbidity and mortality costs. At Murphy's average valuation of $4 million per life, the 560,000 individuals who will die from cancer this year result in losses in trillions, not billions, of dollars.

Five hundred sixty thousand of our fathers, mothers, brothers, sisters, neighbors and friends—that's approximately the same number of men and women who served in Operation Desert Storm. Imagine the reaction if General Norman Schwarzkopf had announced that no Americans sent to the Gulf had survived. Then imagine that that happened every year! That's the impact that cancer should have on all of us.

The approximately $3 billion that we will invest in cancer research in 1999 only allows the NCI to fund about 28 percent of approved research grants; 72 percent go unfunded because of a lack of resources. In the 1970s, the National Cancer Institute could fund 60 percent of these grants. Mr. Chairman, it is clear that we are not advancing as quickly as we should toward victory in this nation's war on cancer.

When President Nixon announced that war in 1971, his intention then was to produce a cure within a decade—just as President Kennedy's earlier goal of putting a man on the Moon had been achieved in less than ten years. We all thought it would work. After all, President Roosevelt had declared war on polio in 1938, and 17 years later, we produced the Salk vaccine. My family knows something about polio because my father had contracted it as a child and I was among the first of the baby boomers to receive the new vaccine. What a simple concept: get a shot and wipe out a disease. Surely we should do the same with cancer.

Then, two years after President Nixon's declaration, my mother-in-law was diagnosed with breast cancer. Four years after that, my father found out he had malignant melanoma. In the late 1970s, following my father's diagnosis, my family began a program of funding cancer research, later expanded and formalized by the Milken Family Foundation. In 1993, I founded CaP CURE to help fight the most commonly diagnosed non-skin cancer in America.

In 1995, I told the National Cancer Summit that General Schwarzkopf, a fellow prostate-cancer patient, believed military lessons should be applied to the war on cancer. "There comes a time," he said, "when you must get on with the battle. You'll never have perfect intelligence on the enemy." The fact is that we have plenty of information for the offensive—we just lack sufficient firepower.

How much firepower do we need? Last fall, as part of THE MARCH . . . COMING TOGETHER TO CONQUER CANCER, I suggested to Senators Connie Mack and Dianne Feinstein, at a hearing of the Senate Cancer Caucus, that the annual federal investment in cancer research be increased to $10 billion. While such a sweeping plan is beyond the immediate purview of this committee, I'd just like to say that a $10 billion investment is less than $40 per American. It is a fraction of the cost of failure—the cost of treating the more than 100 million Americans currently living who are expected to get cancer.

Consider what part of our national income we have spent on the military in wartime, and then consider the fact that an American soldier is more likely to die from cancer than from enemy action. Just as we don't fight guns-and-bullets wars with a 40-hour week, we must recognize that the war against the foreign invader we call cancer is a 24-hour-a-day, seven-day-a-week effort.

A single U.S. company, the Intel Corporation, spends more than twice the government's annual cancer research budget on R&D and capital expenditures: investing in laboratories and research procedures and then investing over and over again as new opportunities for discovery present themselves in subsequent years. Marketplace competition means that the investment is required—not just considered; it is an essential part of the company's success. We should learn from our country's technology leaders and make the same kind of investment in cancer research.

Perhaps it is cooperation and competition from the newly created Department of Defense cancer research projects that has propelled NIH's investments forward in this area. Perhaps it is cooperation and competition from the private sector that has generated rapid results in the National Human Genome Project. With competing companies claiming that they will unravel the human genome quickly, the government project may complete its work a half decade sooner than expected.

Technological advances could propel us further and faster on the road toward a series of cures. Improvements in imaging technology, for example, can help us visualize cancer cells. Adaptations of military technologies can be used to target radiation more effectively. These and thousands of investigations we haven't yet considered—including some that should be declassified from the military—will cost much less than the cost of failure.

An education leader once said, "If you think education is expensive, try ignorance." I would paraphrase that as, "If you think cancer research is expensive, try paying for continued treatment of 100 million Americans."

The 76 million members of the baby-boom generation—31 percent of our population—are turning fifty at the rate of one every seven seconds. As they pass that threshold, their risk of cancer—including prostate cancer—increases. Prostate cancer will affect about one man in six in this country, which means that more than six million boomers could become its victims during the next decades resulting in more than $600 billion in expenditures.

Consider the further economic and social impact of prostate cancer. Take, as an example, the potential impact of the disease on the eight million individuals—including men in uniform and retirees—who receive health care in the Defense Department's worldwide network. It's easy to see, but painful to recognize, that there are—and will continue to be—extraordinary losses in human capital to prostate cancer. It's easy to see, but painful to recognize, that the future liability of prostate cancer is, in fact, in the trillions of dollars. These losses are part of the cumulative skills and experience of men in the workforce—and they are great because prostate cancer most often strikes employees and managers with the longest tenure, men who are in the midst of making their most significant contributions to this country. And the pain will continue—for individuals, families and society—unless we decide to do something about the problem now.

In the six years since my diagnosis, the federal government has invested about $800 million dollars to find a cure for prostate cancer, only about $3,000 for each life lost to the disease. Compare that to the nearly $3 billion our government has wisely appropriated during that six-year period for breast cancer research—a disease that annually claims approximately the same number of lives. Or compare it to the more than $10 billion that the federal government has spent trying to find a cure for AIDS. It's not that breast cancer research or AIDS research gets too much research funding. As long as lives are lost to those diseases, or pain and suffering endured, no amount is "too much." It's just that prostate-cancer research has gotten too little.

Then, Mr. Chairman, in the fiscal year 1999 appropriation, you and your colleagues required a sea change in the prostate cancer research strategy that will, this year, lead to NIH's investment of approximately $175 million. It is an important beginning. On behalf of the more than one-quarter of the families in this country who find or will find a member diagnosed with prostate cancer, we thank you, Mr. Chairman. We also thank the chairman of the full committee, Senator Ted Stevens, and your colleagues on the committee for your leadership.

Still, in the short time I'm speaking today, another American will have died from prostate cancer. That's five men every hour, more than a hundred men every day—almost 40,000 men this year alone. While prostate cancer kills men, its victims are also women—the wives, mothers, daughters, sisters, aunts and friends of those whose lives are cut short—part of the human tragedy of this devastating disease.

That's why it's so encouraging to see that NIH is both increasing and diversifying its investments in prostate cancer research. But, given the aggressive impact of this disease, even this novel, assertive NIH investment strategy may not go far enough—in dollars or research development.

We believe that, as NIH and NCI "ramp up" their efforts to find a cure for prostate cancer, there will be a compelling need to visit with your committee, in the next four years, to ask for more funds for clinical prostate-cancer research. We think important clinical developments are taking place now and, with more funding, will only accelerate. For example, CaP CURE-supported research has already led to more than 70 new treatments that are currently in clinical trials. Among the most promising medical advances are:
   —treatments using viruses programmed to replicate in prostate cancer cells and kill them;
   —new chemotherapies that are successful in stopping the growth of previously untreatable tumors; and
   —novel vaccines that cause patients to mount significant immune responses to their own tumors.

We know that an investment in clinical and translational research makes good business sense. As an example, in the 1980s, experts were predicting that, at the end of this century, American deaths from AIDS would exceed 500,000 annually. While AIDS is still a great human tragedy, this year, about 15,000 people—not half a million people—will die from the disease. We cannot yet celebrate a cure for AIDS and it is wrong to become complacent, but the impact of research breakthroughs through the creation of new treatments has been astounding.

Similarly, we need to accelerate research efforts for prostate cancer. We applaud NCI's creation of QuickTrials and RAID, new programs to hasten new treatments. And we applaud the creation of prevention trials, which could save lives in future generations.

We support NCI's Herculean commitment to collect more than one million men for prevention trials. But we would like to see their similar commitment directed to the collection of one million men—or more—for clinical trials. That fewer than five percent of eligible adults participate in cancer clinical trials—even less in prostate-cancer clinical trials—is staggering, and we'd like to encourage dedicating federal resources and ingenuity to solve that problem.

We would like to see more than five cents of every cancer research dollar dedicated to prostate-cancer research, because we think the value of the investment is already assured. According to the National Prostate Cancer Coalition, which CaP CURE is proud to support and sponsor, at least $500 million could be invested in new and underfunded research areas in 1999. These include:
   —chemotherapies that destroy cancer cells and halt the progression of disease;
   —vaccines and other stimulators of the immune system;
   —anti-angiogenesis therapies that destroy a tumor's nutrient blood supply;
   —differentiation agents that normalize prostate cancer cells;
   —treatments affecting the prostate cancer cell's androgen receptor;
   —promoting apoptosis, or programmed cell death;
   —radiobiology and radiology treatments;
   —tumor molecular biology including the molecular "fingerprinting" of disease;
   —genetics that may help stop the disease at its earliest stages; and
   —nutritional and other alternative therapies that may impede or reverse the progression of disease.

We would like to encourage NIH to reduce barriers related to its grants procedures and encourage a streamlining of the process that would get funds into researchers' laboratories and clinics more rapidly. At CaP CURE, we know it can be done without sacrificing the integrity of peer review.

But there's even more that America can do. While it's beyond the scope of this Committee's work, I believe the Congress should consider tax incentives for research, such as enhanced investment tax credits, R&D credits, and sales of tax-loss carry- forwards. If we have a real war on cancer, then why not issue "cancer war bonds"? Why not extend patent lives, accelerate FDA approvals and authorize direct contracting with corporations for research and development? That kind of public-private partnership helped win World War II and it can win World War Cancer.

I believe in all of these proposals because it's clear to me that we can accelerate science. If we give cancer researchers the same kinds of tools that technology companies employ in accelerating scientific development, we can find a cure faster. That will relieve the suffering of more than 100 million Americans.

We have talented people working on this inside and outside the government. Let's give them the tools and the incentives to finish this job. Let's send a message to our best and brightest young scientists that cancer research is an exciting profession and not—as one CaP CURE-supported scientist was told by his medical-school mentor—"career suicide." Finally, let's show all these dedicated people that we share their sense of urgency.

It is up to you, Mr. Chairman, and your colleagues, to provide and direct the necessary resources to pave the way. We owe this not to ourselves, but to our families and to future generations. We strive to leave our children a nation free from debt and a world free from war—a world that cherishes the sanctity of a single human life. That world must not allow the scourge of cancer to continue. Let us find a cure for cancer now. Let us choose life.

Thank you.

SUMMARY STATEMENT OF JOE TORRE

Senator SPECTER. We turn now to the Manager of the New York Yankees, Mr. Joe Torre. During his 17-year playing career Mr. Torre was named to the All-Star Team 9 times. In 1977 he began his managerial career with the New York Mets. He has managed in Atlanta, St. Louis, and returned to New York to manage the Yankees. Within the past month, after having been diagnosed with prostate cancer earlier this year on March 10 during a routine exam and having undergone surgery, he looks good. The team is winning.

Mr. TORRE. That makes me healthy and look good.

Senator SPECTER. Thank you very much for joining us, Mr. Torre, and the floor is yours.

Mr. TORRE. Mr. Chairman and members of the subcommittee: Again, thank you for having us here.

I am Manager of the Yankees, as of last night anyway. I am also a prostate cancer survivor, also a 4-year survivor of George Steinbrenner, which is not easy. I began managing the Yankees prior to the 1996 season, which was a tough job. After managing several ball clubs coming to the highest profile team in baseball and the toughest media mecca in the world, that was quite a challenge.

In our first 3 years, fortunate and talented, went to the post-season 3 times, won the World Series twice, the first time in 1996, beating the Braves when we were down two games to zero, and then of course last year, winning 114 games and having to validate that by winning the World Series. These were two of the most challenging experiences of my life.

However, none of these challenges have come close to what I dealt with in my battle against prostate cancer. I was diagnosed with prostate cancer this past March. It was discovered during a routine physical in spring training, when my PSA was elevated. A follow-up biopsy confirmed that I did in fact have prostate cancer.

I came out, as did Senator Dole, before I had the surgery. I sort of had no choice. My wife said: See, if you had retired when I asked you to nobody would know about this. But maybe it was the best thing.

After consulting with my doctors, I decided to have surgery to remove the prostate. Dr. Bill Catalona performed the surgery in St. Louis on March 18 and so far everything checks out and I feel wonderful.

A lot of men are diagnosed so late and with the disease so bad that their treatment options are severely limited or nonexistent, and too often the disease comes back.

Mr. Chairman and members of the committee, I thank you for your work you have done to protect men and their families from prostate cancer. But more must be done. When I was initially diagnosed, my first thoughts centered on my family. I have four children, including a 3-year-old daughter named Andrea Rae. This was one of those moments that clarifies personal priorities. The needs and concerns of my family were front and center. Baseball is definitely my life, but being diagnosed with a serious disease makes you realize what is really important.

Fortunately, my family gave me the encouragement that was so crucial to my coping and the initial shock of the diagnosis, as well as the surgery and my ongoing recovery. My wife Ali has given me the unconditional support that I needed and that at the end of the day has made all the difference in my fight against this disease.

During my recovery I also received many letters and phone calls from men who had faced the same challenge. You do not realize how many people are affected until you are on that ball club, I guess.

Also important, members of the Yankee family, led by George Steinbrenner, came to my side during the difficult time. The Yankees, unfortunately, are all too familiar with cancer. This disease in different forms has touched the organization in its history. Babe Ruth lost his life to cancer, last year Darryl Strawberry learned he had colon cancer, and this year Joe DiMaggio died after facing lung cancer and pneumonia.

My close friend Bob Watson, former Yankee general manager, had been battling prostate cancer for several years. He and his wife Carol were outspoken about the need for more research funding when they testified before a Senate committee last year. I look to these people and to my close friends for inspiration and support.

I feel lucky to say that my fight against prostate cancer was a team effort, one that involved many caring family members, friends, fans, and members of the Yankee organization. I know and continue to know that I am not alone in this fight.

Unfortunately, a man dies from this disease every 13 minutes. That is simply too many men and too many wives, daughters, and sons who are devastated by prostate cancer. The toll that this disease takes each day and each year is nothing less than epidemic. While prostate cancer accounts for 15 percent of all cancer diagnosis, only 5 percent of Federal cancer dollars are directed toward prostate cancer research.

A man has a one in six chance of getting prostate cancer in his lifetime if he has a close friend with prostate—if he has a close relative with prostate cancer, his risk doubles. With two close relatives, his risk increases fivefold. Three close relatives, it is nearly 97 percent. Make no mistake, this is a family disease.

As pointed out earlier, the African American community is even more at risk. African American men have the highest prostate rate in the world, 35 to 50 percent greater than the rate of white males, and African American men endure twice the mortality rate.

I am here to tell you that prostate cancer does not discriminate based on age. This is not an old man's disease. About one in four prostate cancer cases strikes a man during his prime working years. I am 58 and the number of men in their forties and fifties who are battling prostate cancer is increasing. Doctors around the country report seeing more aggressive forms of disease in younger men.

These statistics are even more troubling when as we look forward the incidence of prostate cancer is expected to keep rising. Do not forget, as the baby boomer generation ages its risk of prostate cancer, if unchecked, will continue to increase. That is why this hearing is so crucial and why Congress' role in protecting men and their families from prostate cancer will make such a tremendous difference in the lives of millions of Americans.

Congressional action is needed on two key fronts: the first is oversight; the second is providing much needed funding for prostate cancer research. With the ability to hold NIH accountable, Congress can ensure that research dollars and strategies will be effectively directed to break through—to treatment breakthroughs and a cure. Combined with increased research funding, this oversight role brings unprecedented hope to the men and their families who are affected by this disease.

The bottom line is that if we are to mount a serious attack on prostate cancer researchers must have the tools and resources that they need. The NIH plan holds promise for rapid progress toward better treatments and ultimately a cure. But unless this program is adequately funded, it is just a plan on a piece of paper and its promise will remain unrealized.

I commend you, Mr. Chairman, and the other members of this committee, and indeed the entire Senate, for all you have done to accomplish our shared goal of successfully fighting prostate cancer. But I also ask that you do all you can in the coming months and years to provide adequate funding for prostate cancer research. Given that so many lives are at stake, finding a cure for prostate cancer must be a national priority.

With Father's Day just days away, I am happy to be able to spend this holiday with my loved ones. I am also happy to be able to be a spokesman for the CapCURE's Home Run Challenge, its annual week-long effort with major league baseball centered on Father's Day to raise awareness and private sector funding for prostate cancer research.

PREPARED STATEMENT

For too many families, this holiday is a time to remember the fathers, husbands, and brothers who have been lost to this disease. By providing increased research funding, you can stem rising rates of prostate cancer and protect future generations of men and their families from its devastation.

Thank you.

Senator SPECTER. Thank you very much, Mr. Torre.

[The statement follows:]

PREPARED STATEMENT OF JOE TORRE

Mr. Chairman and members of the Subcommittee on Labor, Health & Human Services and Education Appropriations, my name is Joe Torre. I am the manager of the New York Yankees. I am also a prostate cancer survivor.

I began managing the Yankees prior to the 1996 season and immediately faced the significant challenges that come with guiding a high-profile team in a competitive league and the biggest media market in the nation.

In my first three years with the Yankees, we've been fortunate—and talented— enough to appear in post-season play three times, winning the World Championship twice. In 1996, the Yankees overcame a two-games-to-none deficit against the powerful Atlanta Braves in the World Series. And, in 1998, we faced the considerable challenge of validating our American League record of 114 wins in the regular season. These were two of the most-challenging experiences of my life.

None of these challenges, however, has come close to what I dealt with in my battle against prostate cancer. I was diagnosed with prostate cancer this March. After a routine team physical during spring training, I found out that my PSA—Prostate Specific Antigen—level was elevated. A follow-up biopsy confirmed that I did, in fact, have prostate cancer.

After consulting with my doctors, I decided to have surgery to remove my cancerous prostate gland. Dr. William Catalona performed the surgery in St. Louis on March 18th and, so far, everything checks out, and I'm fine. I was lucky, though. A lot of men are diagnosed so late or with disease so bad that their treatment options are severely limited or nonexistent. And, too often, the disease comes back. Mr. Chairman and members of the committee, I thank you for the work you've done to protect men and their families from prostate cancer, but much more must be done.

When I was initially diagnosed, my first thoughts centered on my family. I have four kids, including a 3-year old daughter named Andrea Rae. This was one of those moments that clarifies personal priorities; the needs and concerns of my family were front and center. Certainly, baseball is my life, but being diagnosed with a serious disease like prostate cancer makes you realize what's really important!

Fortunately, my family gave me the encouragement that was so crucial to my coping with the initial shock of the diagnosis—as well as the surgery and my ongoing recovery. My wife, Ali, has given me the unconditional support that I needed and that, at the end of the day, has made all the difference in my fight against this disease. During my recovery, I also received many letters and calls from men who were faced with the same challenge.

Also important, members of the Yankee family—led by George Steinbrenner—came to my side during this difficult time. The Yankees, unfortunately, are all too familiar with cancer. This disease—in different forms—has touched the organization in its history. Babe Ruth lost his life to cancer. Last year, Darryl Strawberry learned he had colon cancer. And this year, Joe DiMaggio died after facing lung cancer and pneumonia.

My close friend Bob Watson, former General Manager of the Yankees, has been battling prostate cancer for several years. He and his wife, Carol, were outspoken about the need for more research funding when they testified before a Senate committee last year. I looked to these people, and to my other close friends, for inspiration and support.

I feel lucky to say that my fight against prostate cancer was a team effort, one that involved many caring family members, friends, fans and members of the Yankees. I knew—and continue to know—that I'm not alone in this fight. I know that, throughout it all, my friends and loved ones were 100 percent behind me.

Unfortunately, a man dies from this disease every 13 minutes. That is simply too many men, and too many wives, daughters and sons, who are devastated by prostate cancer. The toll that this disease takes each day and each year is nothing less than epidemic. While prostate cancer accounts for 15 percent of all cancer diagnoses, only 5 percent of federal cancer dollars are directed toward prostate cancer research.

A man has a one in six chance of getting prostate cancer in his lifetime. If he has a close relative with prostate cancer, his risk doubles. With two close relatives, his risk increases five-fold. With three close relatives, his risk is nearly 97 percent. Make no mistake, this can be a family disease.

The African American community is even more at risk. African-American men have the highest prostate cancer rate in the world, 35 percent–50 percent greater than the rate for white males, and African-American men endure twice the mortality rate.

I'm here to tell you that prostate cancer doesn't discriminate based on age. This is not "an old man's disease." About one in four prostate cancer cases strikes a man during his prime working years, under the age of 65. I am 58 years old and the number of men in their 40s and 50s who are battling prostate cancer is increasing. Doctors around the country report seeing more aggressive forms of the disease in younger men.

These statistics are even more troubling when, as we look forward, the incidence of prostate cancer is expected to keep rising. Don't forget, as the baby boom generation ages, its risk of prostate cancer, if unchecked, will continue to increase. That's why this hearing is so crucial and why Congress's role in protecting men and their families from prostate cancer will make such a tremendous difference in the lives of millions of Americans.

Congressional action is needed on two key fronts: the first is oversight; the second is providing much-needed funding for prostate cancer research. With the ability to hold NIH accountable, Congress can assure that research dollars and strategies will be effectively directed to treatment breakthroughs and a cure. Combined with increased research funding, this oversight role brings unprecedented hope to the men and their families who are affected by prostate cancer.

The bottom line is that if we are to mount a serious attack on prostate cancer, researchers must have the tools and resources that they need. The NIH plan holds promise for rapid progress toward better treatments and ultimately a cure. But unless this program is adequately funded, it's just a plan on a piece of paper and its promise will remain unrealized.

I commend you, Mr. Chairman, the other members of this committee and, indeed, the entire Senate for all you have done to accomplish our shared goal of successfully fighting prostate cancer. But I also ask that you do all you can in the coming months and years to provide adequate funding for prostate-cancer research. Given that so many lives are at stake, finding a cure for prostate cancer must be a national priority.

With Father's Day just days away, I'm happy to be able to spend this holiday with my loved ones. I am also happy to be able to be a spokesman for CaP CURE's "Home Run Challenge," its annual week-long effort with Major League Baseball, centered on Father's Day, to raise awareness and private-sector funding for prostate cancer research. For too many families, this holiday is a time to remember the fathers, husbands and brothers who have been lost to this disease. By providing increased research funding, you can stem rising rates of prostate cancer and protect future generations of men and their families from its devastation.

Thank you.

Senator SPECTER. The situation is this. We will arrive right at the conclusion of the first vote and they should start the second vote unless there are stragglers. Senator Dole knows that better than anyone. But we should be able to return here within 10, 12 minutes, and I think it would be useful if we pursued the subject of how we stimulate public awareness and funding.

So we will recess for just a few minutes.

[A brief recess was taken.]

Senator DOLE. You did a good job.

Senator SPECTER. We will resume the hearing. Thank you, Senator Dole. That was a pretty good job, was it not, taking two votes and back in about 15 minutes. While we were gone, Senator Stevens and I held an informal conference en route. We talked to Senator Roth on the floor. Senator Stevens wants to go easy on that.

Let me yield to Senator Stevens for whatever he thinks ought to be said.

Senator DOLE. Roth has been there, too, yes.

Senator STEVENS. Mr. Milken, we have conferred with the chairman of the Finance Committee about the concept of cancer bonds and we will pursue that. It is a good suggestion. It needs to be defined, but if there is a jurisdictional problem there with regard to Appropriations and Finance we will try and work that out.

Senator SPECTER. Well, let us start there, Mr. Milken. You mentioned the idea of bonds, but I would like to for a few minutes to try to explore ways we can get extra funding and how we can stimulate the interest of the American people in the subject. When Joe Torre and Bob Dole and Mike Milken talk about it, people focus on it. It is a step in the right direction.

We have talked about a number of proposals. Senator Hatfield and Senator Harkin and I were co-sponsors on legislation which had proposed a 1 percent fee on all medical insurance that was written, on the theory that if that was dedicated to research, biotechnical research, that it would cut down the cost of payments that insurance companies would have to make for health delivery. That legislation had never gotten too far.

As I had said earlier, there has been a sense in the Congress to double NIH funding and increase cancer research funding, but when it comes to voting for it the votes have not been there. So what Senator Harkin and I have had to do—and he could not be with us today—is to take our overall budget, which impacts on education programs and drug programs and other health programs and worker safety—we have three Departments, the Department of Labor, the Department of Education, and the Department of Health and Human Services. But we have established the priorities to carve out $2 billion more last year.

That is a very difficult thing to do. We really would like to do it again this year, but I do not know that that is going to be possible, depending on where we come out on the caps.

But Mr. Milken, go into a little bit more detail about how you would suggest structuring the bond program. We are off to a good start with your, was it, a $50 million pledge or $50 billion to get it started?

Senator DOLE. Billion.

Mr. MILKEN. I would like to be able to pledge $50 billion, but I will have to start with $50 million.

Senator SPECTER. That is a pretty good start, Mr. Milken.

Mr. MILKEN. I think the issue there of how do you raise capital to invest in this effort on cancer—one of the real forefronts of our effort for solution, not just of cancer problems but all medical problems, are biotech companies. As I stated earlier, they invested last year in R&D $7.5 billion to try to find cures for medical problems and they collectively lost $2.5 billion. They cannot use the losses that they are achieving.

I know the Governor of New Jersey and others have thought about it from the States' standpoint of allowing them to sell their tax loss carryforwards, something we have allowed other companies to do in the past 30 years, if they redeployed that back into medical research or cancer research. That would enable them to reinvest more, and they are on the forefront of the work that is going on, and this would be a private sector initiative where they would invest their own capital.

Investment tax credits, which have gone into effect many times in the past 30 years in our country when we wanted to encourage people to buy computers or automobiles; we obviously have that opportunity if people do cancer research, saying this is a priority of the government from that standpoint also.

Cancer bonds, I think many of us would be very happy to buy low interest rate government bonds that can be deployed into cancer research in some joint efforts, as Senator Stevens has suggested, to get more capital flowing where it would be matched by both the private industry and the public sector. I think the public-private partnerships in our country's history—the recent landing on Mars last year, a partnership between NASA and other government agencies and Lockheed Martin Marietta and others, was at a cost of less than 10 percent of what the cost was of the first landing we had on Mars and was managed by the private sector.

So I think the ability to interact with one another—there is, and I am sure Dr. Varmus and Dr. Klausner know far better than I, there are significant restrictions on the NIH and the NCI's ability to interact with private industry, and I think one should take a look at those restrictions in interaction.

I think we only have to look today to particularly Silicon Valley to see the benefits to our country through developments where Stanford University and the University of California-Berkeley particularly encouraged interaction between university science centers and private industry, and the benefits that have flowed to our entire country.

Senator DOLE. Mr. Chairman, if I could add a note there, I think in addition to how we raise the capital, we need to raise the awareness of the problem, particularly with men. I mean, men do not see their doctors on a regular basis as most women do. Men do not get annual checkups, and you can have all this research and all these new things happening, but you still have to educate the men to see a doctor.

That is one thing we have been trying to do in a narrower sense, but I think there needs to be a focus on men's health issues and to find people like Joe and Michael and others willing to work together to get the word out, because each of us touch a different group.

I know I talked to the American Foundation for Urological Disease. They have a representative here this morning. They have had thousands of phone calls based on an advertisement that I have done, and taken a little heat on it from the media that is not too bright. They are not here today, but in any event.

Senator SPECTER. They just turned off the cameras.

Senator DOLE. That is all right. [Laughter.]

But it is a serious problem and there are serious consequences. It affects millions and millions of people, whether it is prostate cancer or heart disease or diabetes or whatever it is. Men do not go to the doctor. I do not know—this would all be helpful, of course, if they understand there is a better way to treat things. Maybe they would be more apt to go.

But I think that is an underlying problem that we need to address. A lot of that can be done in the private sector. It is being done by General Schwartzkopf. But Michael Milken started, really, and Joe Torre and others, Senator Stevens, people who have gone public, once they have had the radiation, surgery, whatever, in this area—and I am certain there are others out there who would be willing to help in a broader sense when it comes to men's health.

Mr. MILKEN. Men are very shy, as Senator Dole said, and we have a lot to learn from women. Obviously, Mother's Day comes first in the year, and Mother's Day did come first. Actually, prostate cancer has benefited tremendously from the activism of women, who have dragged their husbands, their fathers, their brothers, their friends, their neighbors. I think the breast cancer movement has served as a great role model for many of the people working in prostate cancer today.

Senator SPECTER. Senator Stevens.

Senator STEVENS. Well, I am interested in pursuing the funding problem. My basic problem as chairman of the Appropriations Committee is we live under caps, absolute limits of expenditures, and there just is no additional money to allocate to this subcommittee. It is going to be one of great challenges of the Congress to be able to fund the whole Labor, Health and Human Services Subcommittee without getting into what we call a train wreck as far as the whole process is concerned with the administration.

My mind goes off on another rabbit trail, and that is if you look at this all cancers combined chart that we have obtained and see that Alaska Native and American Indians, with an incidence of cancer in excess of those of black people, enter in with the black Americans and the Alaskan Natives and put those together, then add in the white Americans, you find that the total of those, of the people who originate in the North American continent, is about ten times that of those who have come to this country from other nations.

There has got to be some environmental research here beyond just medical research to locate that. Up my way, when the mining community wants to find a mineral they start taking people to analyze the water, to see where those trace elements come from, and you just keep going back the tributaries into little streams and, guess what, pretty soon you have got a good indication of where the central lode is. But I do not think we are doing that on this. We are concentrating right now on medical research, and I would like to see more money put into the environmental research on this continent to find out why this is.

But I do believe that we have got—Mike, you have got some great ideas. And Bob, you have been prostate cancer pin-up boy. Without you, we probably would not have had a lot of this recognition we have got right now.

Senator DOLE. I have had a lot of pins stuck in me.

Senator STEVENS. Well, I remember a friend of mine, a good friend of mine, when I held a little meeting at home on the procure concept, talking to people, men who might be interested in this, after I had my surgery, a great friend of mine took me aside and said: Ted, you are wrong; you should not talk—men do not talk about these things; do not talk about this.

I said: You have got to be wrong. The problem is the complications from not knowing are worse than knowing.

Senator DOLE. I think Joe discovered that, too.

Mr. TORRE. There is no question, and the PSA has been our best friend. I will tell you, when Dr. Catalona took out my prostate, he said he held it in his hand and he said he did not see anything wrong with it. So if it was not for the blood test it would have been years down the road before it was discovered with the digital exam and other means. And by that time who knows where it would have gone, because I had an aggressive form of cancer.

Senator STEVENS. I am like you. After it was taken out, I demanded a slice of it and I turned it over to one of my great friends who is a pathologist and said: Was that really cancerous? He came back and said it was really cancerous; you got it just in time. A lot—maybe other people are not that skeptical, but the problem of having that type of operation is an enormous one. But the results I think warrant it. The three of us know that. Mike has got another course.

Mr. MILKEN. I think there is two elements you have raised here, Senator: one, environment and nutrition. The NCI is focused, I believe, on trying to collect up to a million men for prevention trials to measure that. We would also like to see if we could get a million men who have been diagnosed in just the last 6 years with prostate cancer into clinical trials, not just prevention trials.

But as you know, during the cancer march last September we did attempt, and successfully with support, and both of you joined us for lunch, to have a non-fat vegetarian lunch, and we were able to get it on the menu in the Senate Dining Room as a starter.

We have been a little remiss, but Doctors Varmus and Klausner have embraced the concept of maybe reducing the level of fat in the NCI's own dining room if you go down there in the cafeteria. So I think there is a lot of opportunities to focus on what we have learned today and bring that as a potential, using nutrition.

But I think the overriding element in terms of your allocation of funds and the difficulty I think is just bridging the gap of a couple years here. It is only a matter of time before the American people realize how little money has been spent on cancer research. It is only a little time before they realize that we have spent twice as much on the Gulf War as we have on all cancer research in this country in the last 28 years. In an 8-month Gulf War, we decided we could get the resources and allocated it, the world could.

In our efforts that we decided we needed to have a commitment to Yugoslavia and the former parts, that will eventually exceed by a far amount. And the efforts in Somalia exceeded the amount we have spent on cancer research.

So anything in life is a question of allocation of resources. But with 100 million Americans projected to be diagnosed with cancer who are currently living, at some point they will ask themselves for a reallocation. I doubt if the 48 Senators who voted against it will be able to vote that way. Whether that is 2 years away or 1 year away, I do not know, but it is not that far away. And I think the cancer march, the 600 cancer organizations that were here last September, were a clear message that there is an interest here.

When you realize we spend 1 percent of the Federal budget on the NIH to provide health and a healthy future for the people of this country, we might decide we need to spend more than 1 percent of our budget on that area.

Senator STEVENS. Mike you have got a point. I do not dispute that. But of the 13 subcommittees we have got, only one of them will—only one of them will be the same as the funding for 1999 in the year 2000, and that will be Defense, but just barely. In this year, with an agricultural problem, a real disaster in some places, and now with the Kosovo incident taking on a longer proportion, with Bosnia still being there, and Iraq, the problem in Iraq, and with higher alerts in South Korea, we cannot take any more money from defense.

I really do not know where we can get it. I think I am the strongest supporter of what you want to do, but we are doing some other things. For instance, do not forget what we are doing at Walter Reed. We are building a baseline now, whether you know it or not. Military people, men and women, get their annual physical. We are starting to track that over a period of years. We will track that, and we will try to get some more information as detectives look at it, where those people were from, what their backgrounds were. And we are getting more and more incidence of both breast cancer and prostate cancer in the military as a result of the tests that they are taking. We will keep that record going for a series of years and perhaps it will help solve some of these problems we are worried about.

But I tell you, I do not know where the money is going to come from in terms of meeting the necessity to have increased money. And I believe it. That is why I want to explore that cancer bond issue concept. And I do believe the public wants to do that.

If we could put up the money, if we could put up the cancer bonds and get the money in for the next two or three fiscal years, it is my opinion that by the time the baby boomers have retired we will have had such progress that we would reduce the cost of Medicare and Medicaid in that generation, the largest generation in the history of the United States.

So if anyone else has any ideas—it is a grand idea. We have talked about it before, but I think it is time we really pushed it now, because there is no question we have reached the limit of our current budget in terms of this war on cancer. We have got to find some additional money and dedicate it to research, and I would welcome your suggestions.

But I do thank all of you—I have got to go—for what you have done. And Joe, maybe we ought to make you—you have done such a good job winning the World Series, maybe you ought to take on the task of being the chairman of that bond drive.

Thank you very much.

Senator SPECTER. Thank you, Senator Stevens.

Well, thank you very much, Senator Dole, Mr. Torre, Mr. Milken. I think this was very useful, a lot of focus of attention. I know the media will be glad to pick up all of Senator Dole's comments, especially his complimentary comments.

But we will continue to work on it. This subcommittee has not given up on the effort to increase the funding very substantially to NIH. If we can sharpen our pencils to a fine enough point, we are going to try to find $2 billion. And we will pursue these tax ideas.

We get more work done in the well of the Senate, as Senator Dole can comment, with bringing the issue up to Senator Roth, chairman of Finance. He is receptive. We cannot pass any bills on taxes out of this committee, but we are going to pursue it.

There is a lot of determination in what you men have said here today and what the doctors have said that will aid us in that effort. Thank you all very much.

Senator DOLE. You know, they did unveil a stamp in Philadelphia—I was up there a couple weeks ago—a prostate cancer stamp, so it gets back to the awareness. There are a lot of things happening out there that make men aware of it. I think Joe—probably all the baseball players will know about it. That will help, too, because they have got a lot of friends, celebrity status, and men will listen.

Mr. TORRE. But I think Senator Dole's point, one more second about getting examinations, letting men know that it is not a death sentence if you get this thing early and they should not be afraid of taking a physical and taking a blood test, because the blood test does not hurt at all, as long as you turn the other way, and it is very treatable if it is gotten in the early stages. That is what the PSA has done for you.

CONCLUSION OF HEARING

Senator SPECTER. Thank you all very much for being here, that concludes our hearing. The subcommittee will stand in recess subject to the call of the Chair.

[Whereupon, at 11:37 a.m., Wednesday, June 16, the hearing was concluded, and the subcommittee was recessed, to reconvene subject to the call of the Chair.]

○

APEX
TP_CF
9780160602047